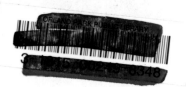

❨ Facing and Fighting Fatigue

Facing and Fighting Fatigue

A Practical Approach

Benjamin H. Natelson, M.D.

Yale University Press ❪ New Haven & London

Published with assistance from the foundation established in memory of Philip Hamilton McMillan of the Class of 1894, Yale College.

The information and suggestions contained in this book are not intended to replace the services of your physician or caregiver. Because each person and each medical situation is unique, you should consult your own physician to get answers to your personal questions, to evaluate any symptoms you may have, or to receive suggestions on appropriate medications.

The author has attempted to make this book as accurate and up-to-date as possible, but it may nevertheless contain errors, omissions, or material that is out of date at the time you read it. Neither the author nor the publisher has any legal responsibility or liability for errors, omissions, out-of-date material, or the reader's application of the medical information or advice contained in this book.

Designed by Rebecca Gibb. Set in Minion type by Keystone Typesetting, Inc. Printed in the United States of America by Vail-Ballou Press, Binghamton, New York.

Library of Congress Cataloging-in-Publication Data
Natelson, Benjamin H.
Facing and fighting fatigue : a practical approach / Benjamin H. Natelson.
p. cm.
Includes bibliographical references and index.
ISBN 0-300-06848-4 (cloth : alk. paper). — ISBN 0-300-07401-8 (pbk. : alk. paper)
1. Fatigue. 2. Chronic fatigue syndrome. I. Title.
RB150.F37N39 1998
616'.0478—dc21
97-30094
CIP

A catalogue record for this book is available from the British Library.

The paper in this book meets the guidelines for permanence and durability of the Committee on Production Guidelines for Book Longevity of the Council on Library Resources.

10 9 8 7 6 5 4 3 2 1

To those of you for whom fatigue is an everyday problem, in the hope that this book will give you ideas for coping.

To my colleagues at the Pasteur Institute and French friends in Paris, who encouraged me to make this book a reality.

To my family, for making me sensitive to the needs of the ill, and to my patients, for convincing me that help is *always* possible.

❴ Contents

⟪ Preface

Fatigue, exhaustion, malaise; wiped out, sleepy, tired, zonked. . . . No matter what the language, the number of words that describe fatigue makes it evident that everyone is aware of the feeling. How to decide whether fatigue is a normal part of life or something more significant is less obvious.

It is my intent in this book to provide knowledge about the causes of fatigue—both the kind that everyone experiences and the kind that is generated by illness—and about the ways to deal with this disturbing symptom. Thus, my goal is to translate a rather intuitive concept into a definition that makes sense to the reader and can be used, when necessary, to combat the fatigue.

For the person who experiences fatigue only at the end of a twelve-hour day or after a long day on the ski slopes, an understanding of the biology involved will suffice to allow that individual to awaken next day feeling refreshed. This book will be of interest to such a person, but it is aimed primarily at the more than 10 percent of the population for whom fatigue is a frequent problem, often of many months' duration. You are the people to whom despite taking the commonsense "cures," fatigue remains a constant companion. You will learn the reasons for your fatigue and understand whether your problem is one of simple tiredness or whether it crosses over into disease—to the illness known as chronic fatigue syndrome. Regardless of your location on the fatigue spectrum, clearly you need other ways to deal with your problem.

My desire to inform you about these tactics is a major reason why I wrote this book. The methods will range from advice you might have thought to give yourself to suggestions that will be new to you. By understanding what fatigue is and what causes it, you will be able to separate truth from fiction, for example in magazine ads that promise you new pep and energy. I will also explain the doctor's problem in dealing with someone complaining of fatigue and suggest ways to break the impasse between you and a doctor who acts as if he or she has no time for you. I will talk about the role of sleep in producing fatigue and suggest how you can improve the quality of your sleep. A number of self-help techniques can help lessen your fatigue, and I will review the medicines and ancillary techniques used in 1997 by the best doctors to treat severe fatiguing illness. For those of you with severe and chronic fatigue, Chapter 10 gives some tips to help cope with your illness.

To those of you whose fatiguing illness has limited your life so severely that you cannot work and need help doing routine daily activities, let me say that I am sure frustration is part of your life: frustration with feeling sick, frustration at not being able to find an understanding doctor, frustration at not being able to find "the" answer. Indeed, your frustration may be one reason why you are reading this book. As you well know, there is no simple cure for severe and long-lasting fatigue, or you would have found it by now. In my opinion, books that provide a simplistic answer are of little value. They may attract a lot of attention, but a few months later a new volume appears and the next fad is launched. My tactic is different: it is to tell you what is known and to suggest ways that help—but unfortunately do not cure. My experience with many hundreds of patients tells me that my approach is helpful and generates a map—albeit crude—of the road to wellness. Knowledge is empowering; it will, I hope, reduce your frustration.

As I start this book, I am recovering from a long transcontinental flight, whose consequence is nearly always jet lag—an acute and self-limited cause of fatigue. Jet lag is one of the surest ways to induce the sort of severe fatigue and confusion about which patients with fatiguing illness complain.

Unless fatigue is excessive, each of us has derived a personal strategy for doing what is necessary to keep on going despite feeling exhausted. This book is written for those who do not have such a strategy, or whose fatigue is excessive and/or accompanied by other symptoms. More often than not, there is a "cure" for your fatigue; even when no such cure exists, you can be helped to manage your fatigue.

I am grateful to many who assisted in the genesis of this book. Dr. Gudrun Lange helped to make Chapter 4 more accessible to the reader, and Dr. Simon Wessely provided citations of articles on chronic fatigue syndrome in medical journals written in languages other than English. David Shannahoff-Khalsa taught me something about kundalini yoga—a lesson I took to heart in Chapter 7. The advice and comments of Dr. Margaret Chesney made Chapters 8 and 9 a lot better the second time around. Dr. Dan Clauw clarified the thinking of rheumatologists for me, especially about fibromyalgia. And Dr. Richard Podell improved my Summing Up in Chapter 13.

1 ❁ Definitions and Prevalence

Fatigue is a concept that we all recognize and understand—until we try to define it. One unambiguous fact is that if we have problems sleeping, fatigue will inevitably follow. It is possible to study fatigue naturally by keeping people awake. The results will be excess fatigue, loss of vigor, increased irritability, feelings of demoralization, even muscle achiness. But simply feeling fatigue is not the same as being able to explain what it is.

A number of definitions exist. One commonly used medical dictionary defines fatigue as "that state following a period of mental or bodily activity characterized by a lessened capacity for work."[1] A similar way of defining fatigue is as a "condition of reduced functional capacity that occurs as a consequence of work and dissipates with rest."[2] These definitions generate immediate problems. In the vast majority of instances, the work gets done despite the fatigue. Most of us are experts at what we do, so for our particular jobs only major problems will cause us to be so tired that we perform those jobs poorly.

Serious problems with fatigue are seen only in rather rare situations. One well-known and unfortunate example is shift workers. Industrial accidents occur much more frequently during night shifts than during day shifts, and fatigue is the direct reason. Most shift workers do not really alter their biological clock, but instead try to maintain a normal social schedule despite working nights. This state of affairs can produce profound fatigue with dangerous consequences. Think of how you felt the last time you flew to Europe or Hawaii, and imagine how you might feel if you had to do so every other day. This is the same sort of situation (of course made worse by the travel involved) that most shift workers undergo. Fatigue is the obvious consequence.

None of the definitions of fatigue permits easy measuring. Although most people's jobs require that they produce a product in a timely manner, the path the individual follows to get his or her work done is very hard to analyze; the rate of making mistakes is much easier to study. But because major mistakes are rare in most people's jobs, the way mistakes are made also becomes hard to study. We are left with the fact that fatigue is a subjective experience not easily measured by objective methods.

Those of us who are interested in understanding fatigue better by developing some objective measure have to leave the workplace and enter the laboratory. There we can develop tasks for people, monkeys, or mice. The tasks must have one thing in common: they must be boringly repetitive (like some factory work) so that the work can be done quickly and without much concentration, and so that the time it takes to do the job correctly can be measured. That time gets longer as fatigue sets in, even when mistakes are not being made. The subject has to stop to think whether he or she is doing the right thing.

Studying fatigue in the laboratory, however, lacks the element of motivation. Here is where human differs from mouse. A researcher can do almost nothing to keep a mouse motivated; when it is fatigued, it sleeps—even if this means it will fall into cold water. For human and for monkey, on the other hand, motivation to stay awake does exist. Laboratory studies of human fatigue, then, are possible. They do, however, require round-the-clock staffing, so they are extremely expensive. Good reasons for studying the monkey! I with my colleagues in the Neurobehavioral Unit at the East Orange (N.J.) Veterans Administration Medical Center have been working on experimental models of fatigue in the laboratory over the past seven years.

The monkey is the one laboratory animal that can be taught to do the sorts of task used to evaluate children with learning disorders. Furthermore, the monkey can be taught to perform those tasks like a factory worker, so that one miss in two hundred trials per day is a rare event. Instead of getting paid at the end of the day or at the end of the week, as would the factory workers, the monkeys get paid each time they do their task correctly. Each payoff is a morsel of food. We have constructed our experiments so that the total amount of food each monkey earns is more than the amount the monkey would take if the food were freely available. When we arranged that the monkey had to do the job correctly twice before receiving the food, we learned to our amazement that the monkey would work nonstop for as long as three days. And this is not because the animal is hungry; he gets more food each twenty-four hours than he would have if he had worked only a ten-hour shift. For some reason, the prospect of getting more food than usual is enough to make a monkey work without stopping. As you might expect if you had to work nonstop for three days, fatigue sets in. Since the monkey is well practiced at the task, he initially does not make mistakes, but he does take longer to reach the food payoff. By the night of the second day, however, the monkey begins to make mistakes. Thus, we have a model of fatigue in a self-motivated nonhuman primate. Unfortunately, these studies are just beginning, so a scientific understanding of fatigue remains in the future. At least for the next couple of years, we must still define fatigue by means of a person's subjective complaint.

That complaint is surprisingly common. In fact, it is among the ten most common problems that bring patients to their doctor—in 1985, for nearly 1 percent of Americans.[3] Just how much of a problem fatigue produces is again a question of definition. One study of 3,938 college undergraduates asked five brief true-false questions about energy, severity of fatigue, and effect of fatigue on school performance, mood, and relations with other people.[4] Seven percent of men and 11 percent of women in the group fell into a "tired" group who answered "true" to at least four of the questions. Apparently, youth is no antidote to fatigue!

This study tells us a number of things: first, fatigue is a characteristic shared by all humans and resembles other characteristics such as height and weight and differs from other states such as cancer or the ability to become pregnant, which occur in only some humans; second, fatigue is common and can resemble personality traits such as cheerfulness or pessimism in that it can exist early in life and presumably last a lifetime; and third, it is a problem for women more often than for men. Indeed, regardless of whether a study has been performed in France, England, or the United States, fatigue is approximately 50 percent more common in women than in men.[5]

Furthermore, our study provides clues to who is susceptible to fatigue. Tired students were three to four times more likely to have mild depression than students whose answers to the questionnaire placed them outside the tired group. Similarly, tired students reported feeling more stressed and showed more evidence of being stressed. These "risk factors" for fatigue appear also in other studies; we will see them again in later chapters of this book. Characteristics specific to you, it seems, may make you more susceptible than others to fatigue.

Different risk factors for fatigue or tiredness exist in people otherwise healthy; physical inactivity, smoking, and alcohol use correlate with fatigue.[6] Thus, if you are physically inactive and out of shape, having to hurry up two flights of stairs will make you more out of breath and subsequently more fatigued than if you are essentially a physically active person. Obviously, one's sensitivity to alcohol is critical. A big lunch, or even a small one, accompanied by a martini or half a bottle of wine is probably the most common cause of acute fatigue that any of us experiences. Meals themselves are a major cause of daytime sleepiness, although as with other things in life, the soporific effect of eating at midday varies from person to person. A friend who works with me has a real problem with sleepiness after lunch. When he comes to work, he gives me the following instructions: "If you are planning a business lunch, give me the bulk of work that you want me to do in the morning—or, better yet, forget lunch completely." If we add alcohol to my friend's business lunch, he would have to be in another culture, where siestas are permitted, in order to survive. In this very specific example of what can produce acute fatigue, susceptibility again varies from person to person. Applying this knowledge to prolonged bouts of fatigue, and figuring out how to use these facts to lessen fatigue, will take additional thought.

A final risk factor for fatigue is low blood pressure—in the United States, considered to be desirable. But a survey of symptoms correlated with low blood pressure found that fatigue and dizziness occurred much more often in people with low blood pressure than in those with normal or high pressure.[7] This association was strongest in women under age 50. In other cultures, such as Germany, low blood pressure is considered to be a medical problem and is treated by medicines to elevate the pressure. Unfortunately, no one has tested the impact of such treatments so low blood pressure is not treated in this way in the United States. For some people low blood pressure is associated with symptoms ranging from fatigue while standing, to the feeling of lightheadedness, or even a tendency to faint. We will consider simple treatments for people who have low blood pressure producing symptoms later in this book.

The growing interest in understanding fatigue and the problems it causes has begun to show itself in the form of population studies. In these medically based opinion polls, large numbers of people are asked questions about how they feel in general and about feelings of fatigue in particular. In one such study, nearly half of the more than thirty thousand people polled provided information.[8] Over 18 percent reported substantial fatigue lasting at least six months, but only 5 percent of the group reported fatigue to be a serious problem (in that it was present at least 50 percent of the time). This severely fatigued group included nearly twice as many women as men. When asked the reason for their fatigue, the majority of respondents cited work, family, or lifestyle problems. The next most frequent cause was thought to be anxiety or depression. Rather than being the marker for a disease that is not a normal part of human experience, like cancer, apparently fatigue can be a normal part of human experience and biology. The authors saw fatigue as similar to alcohol consumption, in that it produces serious medical problems only when extreme.

Studies like these in the general population are helpful in identifying fatigue as a common problem, but how often is it severe enough that it makes someone decide to check with a physician? One study reviewed the complaints of a thousand patients cared for by doctors-in-training over a three-year period at Brooke Army Medical Center in San Antonio.[9] More women were in the group with symptoms than were in another group with no symptoms. Fatigue of short duration was the second most common complaint (after chest pain) and occurred in about 8 percent of these patients. All fatigued patients received thorough medical evaluations, but no cause for the fatigue was found in two-thirds of the group. The current state of knowledge of medical causes is low and, as I will show later, this fact generates problems in communication between the fatigued patient and the doctor.

People come up with different potential causes of their problem. One British study found that subjects attributed their fatigue equally to physical and nonphysical causes.[10] Physical causes such as anemia, diabetes, recent operation, or infection are among the most common reasons for fatigue and will be discussed in more detail later. Other attributions include social factors—usually shiftwork or overwork—and emotional problems such as anxiety, stress, or depression. Lack of sleep was a common complaint in 15 percent of both men and women. So this study suggests that fatigue hinges in part on causes—medical, psychological, and situational—that can be treated and even cured.

A number of recent studies have focused on the problem of fatigue seen by primary-care practitioners. How often fatigue emerges as a patient complaint depends on the way the question is asked. Yet, one generalization is clear: more women than men had a problem with this symptom. When patients in a primary-care practice were questioned about having a serious problem with fatigue, nearly a quarter answered that they did. But only about half of this number—about 13 percent—visited a doctor complaining on their own of fatigue, and only half of these—about 7 percent—cited fatigue as the major problem.[11] These studies of fatigue in primary care are particularly interesting because they look beyond the simple complaint of fatigue and try to differentiate patients based on the duration and severity of fatigue plus the presence of other symptoms.

This flurry of interest in the medical community has been generated by the recognition of an entity known as chronic fatigue syndrome (CFS). Although I shall devote an entire chapter to this illness, a brief definition is in order here. It is considered to be an illness characterized by pervasive fatigue that produces significant disability and lasts more than six months. What is not yet clear is whether CFS is just an extreme example of the fatigue that appears to be part of the human condition or whether it is a disease, comparable to cancer or severe infection.

A recent study is instructive.[12] One thousand consecutive patients in a primary-care clinic were examined for the existence of unusual, debilitating fatigue. As we have seen, when patients are asked about the presence of fatigue, many of them answer affirmatively—27 percent, in fact. But two-thirds of this particular group had a medical or psychiatric condition that could explain their problem. The great majority of the remaining patients who said they had debilitating fatigue of at least six months' duration without apparent cause were women. Surprisingly, of the seventy-four patients with this complaint who were available for follow-up testing, two-thirds were not interested in having a careful medical evaluation. Although the reasons were not specified, one real possibility is that, despite checking the appropriate answers on their questionnaires, the patients were not really much concerned about their fatigue—or perhaps they were skeptical that further testing would help them. Only three of the chronic fatigue patients who were willing to be evaluated had the additional symptom picture needed to make the diagnosis of CFS from the definition developed by a group of American researchers.[13] And only one of the three fit the definition perfectly. Because the number of patients with severe and chronic fatigue had shrunk considerably, the exact prevalence of CFS could not be pinpointed, but it was estimated that up to 0.3 percent of the patients going to a doctor's office had CFS.

A second study by the same group, despite a broader population base, had very similar results.[14] Instead of using patients seeking medical care (as in the previous study), the group asked members of a health maintenance organization—regardless of health status—if they suffered from fatigue. Again those complaining of fatigue were more often women, and more than half of them chose not to participate in the study because of insufficient interest or time. Most people in this group were able to attend to their primary responsibilities at home or at work, so their symptoms were probably mild. Again, this unwillingness to participate made it difficult to determine how frequently

CFS occurs, but an estimate of 0.1 percent of this community-based population seemed reasonable. Since not every American goes to his or her doctor on an annual basis, this is probably the best possible estimate based on the original definition of CFS and translates into about 250,000 Americans having CFS at any one time. I use the word "original" because a group of experts subsequently articulated a definition that will be easier to meet.[15] An English group has used this new definition in following up 2,376 patients who went to their doctor for common viral infections.[16] They found that 0.5 percent of the group fulfilled the new definition and had no competing psychological disorder that might cause confusion. This figure is five times larger than that found using the more restrictive definition and translates into more than one million people with this illness in the United States—again mostly women. This is a significant number that has real economic consequences for our nation in terms of health-care expenditures, lost income, and the inability to work. Furthermore, the problem extends to Holland, Canada, Scotland, Australia, and New Zealand—countries where major research teams are working on the problem. Moreover, papers reporting the syndrome in other European countries and in Japan make it clear that CFS is a worldwide problem with worldwide economic ramifications.

It is important to read between the lines here. Different grades or degrees of fatigue exist. There is the fatigue that comes and goes—for instance, when one is under a lot of stress or physically very active. This fatigue disappears with rest or when the period of stress or high activity ends. Then there is the fatigue that follows infection. Infectious mononucleosis is the best example. Mono is an illness that often starts with a severe sore throat, swollen glands, fever, and fatigue. Eventually the sore throat, swollen glands, and fever vanish; the fatigue can be slower to disappear. Ninety-five times out of a hundred, it is gone within six months. But about 5 percent of such patients never get better and eventually are diagnosed as having CFS. We now know that postinfectious chronic fatigue is an entity, thankfully a rare one. I will have more to say about postinfectious fatigue in Chapter 4.

A surprising number of people with no recent history of mono are bothered by fatigue that lasts longer than six months. For some, the fatigue does not produce a major change in their way of life. They have chronic fatigue, but fall in the mild category. Another group of people have severe and long-lasting fatigue.[17] A relatively small portion of this group have other symptoms that allow their doctor to diagnose CFS. Their physician, more often than not while considering that diagnosis, finds a medical or psychiatric cause for the symptoms. Causes generate solutions, and the number of sufferers therefore decreases. Since a surprisingly large number of patients in this remaining group are not interested in learning more about their problem, we can assume that similarly large numbers of the group who have severe chronic fatigue but not CFS also are managing well.

It seems, then, that the vast majority of people with fatigue manage adequately on their own. Either their fatigue is mild or they have learned to live with it. Still, approximately one million Americans have CFS requiring medical help. And obviously millions more who do not have CFS need help in coping with their fatigue and other symptoms. Those of you who fall in these categories need to realize that, in association with your doctor or some other care provider, you *can* reduce your fatigue. It is like stopping smoking. Some can do it on their own; others need help. The important point is that you can be better!

2 ❦ Causes of Fatigue

Every one of us has a time each day when fatigue hits. For the human lark, it is at night; for the human owl, it is early in the day. Regardless of the setting of our biological clock, a basic activity/rest rhythm guides our lives: the sleep/wake rhythm that is regulated mostly by light and dark. Because of the clock-like nature of earth's rotation, a night/day sequence lasts exactly twenty-four hours. Inevitably, a person gets up in the morning, is active, and rests during the night. Nocturnal animals such as mice do the same thing but at opposite times of day.

Inside this overall sleep/wake rhythm, other rhythms exist. Some follow stimuli in the environment—such as a big lunch, or a small lunch but a big martini—while others seem to track the body's own biological clock. Some information exists about changes in the perception of one's energy across the day. One group surveyed the energy levels of a number of groups of volunteers four times during each waking day. The major finding was that regardless of whether the group was healthy or currently suffering from chronic fatigue syndrome, perceptions of vigor were higher in the morning than at other times of day. One difference between patients and healthy volunteers was that the patients consistently felt the least energy late in their waking day, whereas healthy volunteers tended to have their low point soon after lunch. Interestingly, the normal energy pattern of healthy people and CFS patients differs strikingly from that of depressed patients.[1] For those individuals, mood and activity levels are lowest in the morning—rising (if at all) later in the day.

Clearly, biological rhythms of energy and/or fatigue exist, and fatiguing illness or depression can alter these patterns. What other factors can produce fatigue?

Common Causes

The usual causes of fatigue for an otherwise healthy person include those dictated by common sense: poor sleep, excess stress, a personality that tends toward anxiety or toward depression. We need to pay attention to each of these factors because, as we will see, each can be reduced by its own particular prescription.

Poor sleep with resulting fatigue is most commonly caused by the items listed above. Thus, even before you are conscious that you are stressed, you may all of a sudden find yourself waking up repeatedly during the night to look at the time. Stress is your body's response to the pressures in your everyday life, while anxiety and depression can be the ways you as an individual react to stress. Since one person's pressure is another person's pleasure, there is huge variability in what makes stress develop in any one person.

Nervousness

Anxiety or nervousness is a trait that usually is part of one's personality. If you ask people if they consider themselves nervous, they will often tell you spontaneously that they are and have been so for as long as they can remember. So personality is important in determining whether one feels stressed or not. Shy people, for instance, often feel very uncomfortable—that is, feel stressed—when put in social situations where they have to "act properly." Regardless of what triggers it, stress makes itself apparent by producing an upset stomach, a feeling of flush, and a racing heart. The only thing that I know regularly produces such a sensation in me is being late for something important—like a plane to Paris.

The lifetime problem of nervousness that some people inherit is one form of anxiety, but other forms can result from experiences with extremely frightening or emotionally upsetting events. Depending on the severity of the trauma and on factors specific to the individual, some people do not recover from a stressful encounter and instead develop a form of chronic stress. Probably the most common form is known as post-traumatic stress disorder (PTSD). This problem was originally recognized in soldiers in battle who had been exposed to life-threatening situations. Now we know that this disorder is not limited to soldiers, but occurs all too often in civilians. Reports of its occurrence following Iraqi missile attacks in Israel and in women after rape indicate that only one exposure to an extremely stressful event can produce this altered mental state. This form of chronic stress requires professional care, and to date the field of psychiatry has only focused on the psychiatric consequences of exposure to extreme stress. But what about less severe stress; can it also produce permanent changes in feelings and the development of fatigue? What about a car accident? What about an armed robbery? What about a job that you hate? My bet is that less resilient people will develop chronic stress in any of these situations. Although the symptoms may not have the severity of those seen in PTSD, they will probably produce chronic stress, which is commonly manifested by fatigue and nervousness.

Depression and Dysthymia

Depression frequently goes hand in hand with fatigue. Many patients who have depression may not be aware of its existence, for it usually has a slow and insidious beginning. The start of a depressive illness is quite different from the start of a cold or a heart attack, in which you are suddenly besieged by a set of uncomfortable and/or frightening symptoms. There is no clear-cut onset; you just feel a little worse from one day to the next. Identification is sometimes made more difficult by the fact that symptoms that people equate with depression are not always experienced. You do not have to feel blue to be depressed; if you have lost interest in most of the activities that used to interest you, that can indicate the existence of depression. Similarly, if you are sad and disheartened but free of guilt and you never entertain the thought of suicide, you could still be depressed.

From these examples it is obvious that depression can have many faces. Because there are no blood tests and no specific behaviors that are characteristic of depression, psychiatrists have tried to decide by committee what constitutes psychiatric illness. These consensus groups—which decide to agree despite the existence of substantial disagreement—have arrived at lists of major and minor symptoms that are needed for a diagnosis of depression. The symptom lists constitute a "case definition" of depression. In general, the lists fall into two categories, those of typical depression and those of atypical depression.

Major symptoms for typical depression include the presence of depressed mood and markedly diminished interest in most activities most of the day for at least two weeks. In addition, at least four of the following minor symptoms (only three are needed if both major symptoms exist) must have been present for at least two weeks: weight change, altered sleep pattern, agitated or clearly slowed movements, fatigue or loss of energy, feelings of worthlessness or guilt, difficulty in concentrating or indecisiveness, and thoughts of death or suicidal ideation. Thus, if a person had this entire laundry list of symptoms for one week and then felt fine, he or she would not technically be considered to have major depression. Obviously if these symptoms recurred often enough, the doctor would have to put away his textbook, make the diagnosis of depression, and initiate treatment.

Perhaps because I am not a psychiatrist and was never formally taught to think like one, I have a different definition of serious depression. I define it as any symptom or uncomfortable feeling that anti-depressant medication removes. I will explain this in more detail in a later chapter, when I discuss treatment of fatigue. Here I simply want to say that a trial of antidepressant therapy sometimes will have surprising results for a whole range of symptoms such as fatigue, headache, and other sorts of severe pain that are not commonly thought to reflect depression.

Obviously, an all-or-nothing diagnosis like the one used by psychiatrists will leave out a lot of troubled people. To deal with this shortcoming, the consensus group came up with a way of defining the person whose life is filled with despair and doom and gloom—at least that is the way the person believes her life to be (I say "her" because depression is more common in women than men at almost every age).[2] This person is said to suffer from dysthymia, which is defined formally as the existence of a chronic depressed mood lasting at least two years *plus* at least two additional depressive symptoms.

Obviously this plan of providing lists from general categories is one that is oriented toward the practicing doctor, most often to the practicing psychiatrist. Looking over these lists in terms of your own experience, most of you can pretty well know whether you have or have ever had major depression or dysthymia. Others of you will not be so sure. That is where questionnaires are helpful: they do not allow a physician or psychologist to make the clinical diagnosis of depression, but they can identify that a problem with depression exists. So a moderately elevated score would suggest that you are depressed or blue but probably do not have major depression. The higher your score, the greater the possibility that major depression exists.

The questionnaire in Table 1 is one such approach. It has been used by the Center for Epidemiological Study (of the National Institute of Mental Health in Bethesda, Maryland) to study depression, so is

Table 1 A paper-and-pencil method of identifying possible depression

Directions: Circle the number for each statement which best describes how often you felt or behaved this way DURING THE PAST WEEK.	Rarely or None of the Time (0–1 Day)	Some or a Little of the Time (1–2 Days)	Occasionally or a Moderate Amount of Time (3–4 Days)	Most or All of the Time (5–7 Days)
1. I was bothered by things that usually don't bother me:	0	1	2	3
2. I did not feel like eating; my appetite was poor:	0	1	2	3
3. I felt that I could not shake off the blues even with help from my family or friends:	0	1	2	3
4. I felt that I was just as good as other people:	0	1	2	3
5. I had trouble keeping my mind on what I was doing:	0	1	2	3
6. I felt depressed:	0	1	2	3
7. I felt that everything I did was an effort:	0	1	2	3
8. I felt hopeful about the future:	0	1	2	3
9. I thought my life has been a failure:	0	1	2	3
10. I felt fearful:	0	1	2	3
11. My sleep was restless:	0	1	2	3
12. I was happy:	0	1	2	3
13. I talked less than usual:	0	1	2	3
14. I felt lonely:	0	1	2	3
15. People were unfriendly:	0	1	2	3
16. I enjoyed life:	0	1	2	3
17. I had crying spells:	0	1	2	3
18. I felt sad:	0	1	2	3
19. I felt that people disliked me:	0	1	2	3
20. I could not "get going":	0	1	2	3

Source: Used by the Center for Epidemiological Study of the National Institute of Mental Health, Bethesda, Maryland.

called the CES-D.[3] The questionnaire is scored by adding all the points directly except for questions 4, 8, 12, and 16, where the scores are reversed (that is, a score of 3 would be a 0 and a score of 2 would be a 1, and so on). Scores of more than 15 are thought to reflect the presence of some depression, but primarily in people who do not also have medical complaints. In the presence of medical complaints, not until scores are higher than 26 do they start to strongly suggest the existence of major depression.[4]

In contrast to these examples of typical depression, a form of the illness exists which is atypical, meaning that the opposite sorts of minor symptoms are seen. Thus, instead of problems with insomnia, the complaint is one of sleeping too much; instead of the usual loss of weight, patients complain of weight gain. One example of atypical depression is seasonal affective disorder (SAD). The illness is characterized by a seasonal problem consisting of feelings of diminished well-being, lower energy, sleeping more than usual, having less social activity, weight gain, and increased appetite. This problem occurs most frequently in the winter and is commonly known as the winter blues.

The common denominator of all these symptoms—excessive stress, trouble sleeping, anxiety, and depression—is fatigue. Because these problems are so common in contemporary society, they are the leading causes of fatigue. And because of the frequency with which each is seen, they have attracted an enormous amount of attention by clinical researchers in the past decade. A series of effective treatments has been developed, a side benefit of which is the disappearance of fatigue.

Constitutional Fatigue
Before I turn to the medical causes of fatigue, I want to mention what I call constitutional fatigue. Although both my practice and my research activities focus on patients with the new onset of severe and chronic fatigue accompanied by flu-like symptoms, I occasionally see patients who tell me they have been fatigued all their lives. These are people whose every effort has always produced exhaustion and who, because of their constitution rather than by choice, rest as often as possible. Society may view them as lazy, but to me they represent one extreme of a normal distribution which, like height, can range from the extremes of very short to very tall. These people are just very fatigued. By definition, they do not have chronic fatigue syndrome because their fatigue is lifelong. And frequently fatigue is their only problem; that is, they do not have the flu-like symptoms that mark a

patient with CFS. Because of the duration of the problem, the affected individuals often adjust to their disability. They take jobs where rests are possible or where the work-to-vacation ratio is favorable. I believe that such individuals are the way they are because of their brain chemistry. Thus, although they definitely do not have CFS, the treatments for that disorder, being nonspecific and designed to relieve fatigue, may be helpful. I discuss those treatments in Chapters 11 and 12.

Medical Causes

I want now to turn to some of the medical causes of fatigue. Everyone has experienced acute fatiguing illness. The most common example is, of course, the flu. It is a good example because it makes the point that there are many different kinds of fatigue. In contrast to the relatively pleasant fatigue that follows a day of physical activity, the fatigue that accompanies the flu is quite unpleasant; it produces a washed-out, sick feeling that is called malaise. Moreover, it does not come alone. It is accompanied by fever, often a sore throat, achiness in muscles, joints, and head, disturbed sleep, and frequently problems with attention and concentration.

In thinking about medical causes of fatigue, the doctor always has to develop as complete a list as possible of the symptoms that accompany the fatigue. From this symptom list a set of possible causes can be derived. When fatigue has no accompanying symptoms, the chances of finding a cause rise. Certainly the doctor's first concern should be for the symptoms discussed in the first part of this chapter. If there is no evidence of any of those, what should the doctor look for next?

The list is a long one, because fatigue is a frequent complaint in nearly every ailment. But some illnesses occur a lot more often than others. The purpose of this chapter is to lay out the most common examples of illnesses that produce fatigue as a major symptom. Some occur more often than others. Doctors or other health professionals may wonder why I am not including an illness that they worry about. My purpose is not to include every possibility, but rather to give an idea of the sorts of problems that can puzzle even the clever diagnostician.

Common examples of fatiguing illnesses would include anemia, in which the number of oxygen-carrying red blood cells is low. Thus physical activities that would otherwise be effortless take substantial effort and can produce actual breathlessness. Another example might be early heart failure, where the heart is diseased and unable to pump oxygen-laden blood to the organs that require it, thereby producing fatigue and the inability to do what might otherwise be a trivial task.

Another common cause of fatigue lies in decreased thyroid function or hypothyroidism. As with anemia and heart failure, fatigue is an early sign of this disorder. One of the purposes of the thyroid is to maintain the body's resting metabolic activity. When the thyroid is overactive, metabolic activity goes up, the person sweats, can get very nervous, loses weight despite overeating, and develops a fine tremor at the ends of the fingers. When the gland becomes inactive or is destroyed, fatigue, cold intolerance, and weight gain occur. The reasons for an adult's loss of thyroid function are unclear. Sometimes the cause seems to be viral infection. Such an infection may trigger an immune response directed against the organs of one's own body, producing an illness known as an autoimmune disease. Fortunately, this does not happen too often, but a relatively common target for autoimmune attack is the thyroid gland. Autoimmune diseases in general occur more often in women than in men.[5]

The diagnosis of thyroid dysfunction is made rather simply by appropriate blood tests. And despite the continued presence of immune abnormalities, the symptoms that stem from abnormal functioning of the thyroid can be totally removed by appropriate hormonal treatment.

Fatigue is a common symptom of other kinds of autoimmune

diseases as well. On occasion, these diseases can produce serious, often life-threatening medical crises. The principal examples are rheumatoid arthritis and lupus erythematosus, or LE. Because these diseases produce symptoms in muscles and joints, they are classified as rheumatic diseases. "Rheumatic" comes from the ancient word "rheum," the watery material that produces swelling and symptoms in muscles and joints. As with autoimmune thyroid disease, rheumatic diseases occur more often in women than in men.[6] Although fatigue is a common early symptom, severe arthritic complaints—pain, often accompanied by red and swollen joints—suggest some other medical illness. Often, but not always, blood testing can be used to make the diagnosis. In rare instances the blood test never becomes positive; when this happens, the doctor is able to ascertain the presence of autoimmune disorders by the problems they produce over time.

Although some of the medical causes of fatigue that I have mentioned do not occur often, they are the sorts of problems that the physician is best trained to find and diagnose. The reason doctors have difficulty in diagnosing some illnesses more than others is the way they have been taught to think about patients and disease. I will discuss this more fully in Chapter 5. Here it is important to note that the procedures for which the doctor is best trained—careful examinations and lab tests—are usually what are needed to diagnose illnesses such as the ones I have discussed. Unfortunately, other medical conditions are not as easy to diagnose.

Chronic Infection

One of these is chronic infection. The actual site of infection is less important than the fact that the doctor has difficulty in finding it. Examples include chronic sinus or gum infections, both of which can result in fatigue, low-grade fever, malodorous breath, and face pain. These sorts of chronic infections can go undiagnosed for long periods of time. Hidden or covert infections can also occur in a person who has had prior belly surgery. Once a surgeon has had to enter the abdomen, things inside are never the same. One serious consequence can be a small pocket of infection—an abscess. It can produce the same picture of fever and fatigue I have been describing and is very difficult to identify, even when using special body-imaging tests that can show abscesses. Luckily these hidden infections are very rare.

These types of infections are all similar in that they are localized but not obvious. Perhaps the harder problem is the nonlocalized chronic infection. Increasingly common examples of these in the mid-1990s are early acquired immune deficiency syndrome (AIDS), Lyme disease, or tuberculosis (TB). A prominent early sign in each of these diseases is fatigue.

AIDS

The problem for the doctor in each of these illnesses is the diagnosis. Obviously, if the tests come back positive, the diagnosis is made and there is no problem. Unfortunately, a negative result in the case of each illness does not exclude the possibility that the infection exists. For AIDS, there is a period between the infection and the body's response to the infection by making the antibodies that result in a positive test. The physician can deal with this time lag by simply retesting the blood several months after the original negative test. With the risk factors for AIDS changing in the mid-1990s to favor heterosexual transmission of the virus, this test is necessary in any sexually active person who develops the new complaint of fatigue.

Lyme Disease

The problem is more complex when it comes to Lyme infection. In the majority of cases, the diagnosis is straightforward. The elements include a tick bite; a skin rash that looks like an enlarging target; a flu-like illness that can be followed by attacks of red, swollen joints; and problems in the heart or nervous system. If a patient reports the rash (which is in itself diagnostic) and then later medical problems, the diagnosis of Lyme disease is pretty clear whether or not the blood test comes back positive. But many people have no recollection of a tick bite, and unless one looks closely, the rash may be very hard to see. So for some patients, the diagnosis hinges on an abnormal lab test. Unfortunately, an appropriate standardized test does not yet exist. The same individual can test positive in one lab and negative in another, leaving the doctor unsure about the presence of Lyme disease. A second problem—relatively uncommon in the United States—is that you can have the Lyme infection but continue to test negatively on standard laboratory diagnostic tests, because your body does not show the normal immune response to the Lyme bacteria.[7] A final diagnostic problem is that it is possible for a patient to receive what is currently thought to be the correct treatment for Lyme disease but not be cured.[8] Arguments continue to rage in the medical literature about how common this problem is, but a number of researchers have reported that it can and does happen.

Tuberculosis

Diagnosis of tuberculosis is currently going through a revolution. In the past, diagnosis demanded the ability to culture the TB bacteria. The doctor had to be able to obtain a sample of body fluid containing the bacteria. This would be easily done if the patient had active TB in his lungs and was coughing up bacteria-laden phlegm. However, even for this patient a definite diagnosis could take up to several months because the TB bacterium grows very slowly. For patients who did not have active lung TB, diagnosis was a lot harder. The problem seems to be disappearing now, with the development of a new test that checks for the presence of the TB bacteria themselves, even if in very small numbers.[9] By means of a chemical process called the polymerase chain reaction, or PCR, this test uses techniques from molecular biology that rapidly produce millions of copies of a portion of the bacterial cell wall. These pure copies can then be linked to oppositely constructed copies that have been prepared with a tag to allow the paired copies to be visible. This test is being readied for standard use in diagnosing TB. In the not-too-distant future, it probably will also be used for diagnosis in AIDS and Lyme disease.

Sleep Disorders

Another set of disorders that can produce fatigue are those related to sleep. As noted earlier, anxiety, depression, or stress can disrupt sleep. However, sleep is a bodily function that can also be altered by specific brain abnormalities. One study followed the sleep of a group of patients who had had infectious mononucleosis.[10] This starts as a severe viral illness, sudden in onset and associated with severe fatigue, sore throat, fever, swollen glands, diffuse achiness, and problems with concentration and attention. Usually the illness dissipates, for some individuals it lasts only a few weeks, while for others it can last a few months. A small number of patients develop hypersomnia, which is the need to sleep more than ever before in their lives; other symptoms include problems waking in the morning, and occasional confusion or disorientation. These particular sleep studies were remarkably normal except for the fact that the post-mono group slept more than the healthy group. All of the patients had to nap on a daily basis. Unfortunately, the problem did not seem to disappear despite the passage of time. Every one of the twelve patients studied had to modify his life in one way or another, and only four were able to reach their career goals. The concept drawn from this report is that viral infection can somehow change brain function in such a way as to disrupt the restorative powers of sleep. We will recall this possibility when we talk about CFS.

Sleep Apnea

A much more common cause of sleep-related fatigue results from a medical problem known as sleep apnea.[11] I have been careful to label this condition a medical problem and not a disease, because it appears to result from a combination of natural aging and its almost inevitable companion, weight gain. The condition is seen commonly, but more often in men than in women. The presence of obesity marks a major risk factor. The problem is one of sleep-disordered breathing, and the major marker is the presence of snoring. When someone snores, that means that his or her breathing is not normal. The body has two major responses to poor breathing: first, it wakes you up, although only for a moment, and second, a vicious cycle begins. The cycle is characterized by breathing interrupted by heavy snoring, which progresses to periods when the person does not breathe at all.

These periods of sleep apnea can be very dramatic. I have a relative with the disorder. His snoring is so thunderous that we have to put him in the corner of our house that is farthest away from the rest of us. But the snoring is not the worst thing: what is much worse is that when he snores, the thunderous noise can suddenly stop. This happens because he has completely stopped breathing, so that we hear nothing but deathly silence that can last for a full minute—only to be followed by a really loud snore.

The cause of these episodes of sleep apnea is the narrow opening at the back of the mouth to the windpipe. With age and obesity, that part of the body becomes less rigid and the tongue becomes more flaccid. The combination results in the root of the tongue's falling backward to close off the opening to the windpipe. This produces the obstruction that leads to the gigantic snores. As this situation gets worse, the opening to the airway becomes totally blocked and sleep apnea occurs. Sleep apnea results in agitated, interrupted sleep—that is, the person keeps trying to breathe, and tosses and turns until he can get air into his lungs. As can be expected, the outcome of these episodes of interrupted sleep is extreme daytime sleepiness and wakening unrefreshed. An unfortunate set of consequences includes automobile accidents and increased risk for cardiovascular disease.

A report of heavy snoring and periods of sleep apnea from someone in the house is usually sufficient to suggest this problem, but a definitive diagnosis requires the individual to spend a night in a sleep laboratory, where the number of episodes of sleep apnea and the duration of each apneic event are tabulated to determine apnea severity. Two percent of women and four percent of men in the middle-aged work force are estimated to have definite sleep apnea.[12] The entire problem can be effectively cured by the nightly use of a nasal device that pumps room air past the blockage. For the minority of patients whose problem is compounded by enlarged adenoid glands at the back of their throat, which act as an additional blockade of the free flow of air into the lungs, surgical removal of those glands by means of an adenoidectomy can be done with little risk to the patient, and the promise of a cure. Snoring without apnea is annoying, but probably not a serious health hazard. Very often the use of elastic strips across the bridge of the nose (to help open the nasal passages) is effective in reducing snoring. These strips are available in most pharmacies. Also available are mouthpiece-type devices, which limit the motion of the tongue during sleep. The National Heart, Lung and Blood Institute provides a free book called *Facts about Sleep Apnea* (publication number 95-3798; phone 301-251-1222 or fax 301-251-1223).

Restless Legs Syndrome

A second rather common sleep problem relates to leg movements either while asleep or while falling asleep. Moving one's legs while asleep is normal, but sometimes the movements are so strong that they wake up the sleeper. If this occurs repeatedly throughout the night, the result is excessive daytime sleepiness. A variation can occur at the time the person tries to fall asleep. He or she develops a sort of drawing feeling in the legs, which is relieved by moving them; this particular problem is called the restless legs syndrome. The annoying feeling acts like an alarm clock and prevents restful sleep. Medications are available to treat both conditions.

Neurological Problems: Myasthenia and Multiple Sclerosis
The final set of illnesses to be considered in evaluating a patient whose complaint is primarily fatigue comes from my own discipline, neurology. The first and rarer condition is called myasthenia, which means muscle weakness. The illness occurs at two different stages of life. The first is more common in young women, and the second occurs in older people of either gender. The common complaints are weakness and, of course, fatigue. Frequently when the illness occurs in young women, the first complaints have to do with weakness in the face or head—double vision, trouble holding one's head up. To the practicing neurologist these complaints in a young woman can only spell myasthenia. Occasionally the complaint is less specific. One telltale symptom is that the problem gets worse late in the day. So the patient may feel normal when she awakes but develops a lot of fatigue and actual weakness as the day progresses. When the doctor arrives at this diagnosis, his medical training allows him to proceed in such a way as to decide with almost 100 percent certainty whether or not the illness is present. If the tests come back negative, myasthenia cannot be the cause of the fatigue. If the tests are positive, a set of treatments—some surgical and some with medicines—can be utilized.

The last disease that can start with fatigue alone is multiple sclerosis (MS). Perhaps because it too is an autoimmune disease, MS occurs somewhat more often in women than in men. The diagnosis of MS is usually based on a person's complaint of having had several neurological problems such as double vision, weakness on one side of the body, or walking as if they were drunk at different times in their lives. Obviously, no one can make the diagnosis of MS without the passage of sufficient time so that the doctor can see this pattern of symptoms. One study reported that fatigue was very common in patients with the diagnosis of MS.[13] The study, however, did not require a definitive diagnosis of MS by a trained neurologist and did not provide information as to the severity of the disease. Fatigue will accompany any incapacitating illness. The more important question for the doctor is how often fatigue is a problem for those who turn out to have MS but in whom the diagnosis is not clear.

In order to get some information on this question, I turned to a group of patients who definitely had MS but whose disease was often so mild that it could not be recognized without a careful neurological evaluation. Of the nineteen patients I evaluated, only three did not have major complaints of fatigue. And at the time of evaluation, these three patients were almost symptom free. This small study suggests that fatigue is an early and consistent complaint of MS patients. A recent study from Holland supports the point and notes that MS fatigue is not related to depression or to severity of MS symptoms.[14] The fact that MS severity and fatigue do not go hand in hand is rather surprising. Djaldetti and her colleagues in Tel Aviv, using actual muscle testing to assess fatigue in MS patients, found worse fatigue during an MS flareup than during quiescent periods.[15] This study suggests that fatigue after effort may be an ever increasing problem as the MS progresses. Whether or not the new treatments for MS will relieve this persistent problem is not currently known, especially because fatigue and other MS symptoms are unrelated.

The question then remains: How does a physician make the diagnosis of MS in a patient who has not had repeated neurological problems separated from one another by periods of normalcy? Strictly speaking, the diagnosis of MS must await development of this clinical pattern, but the doctor can—if fatigue is a severe problem, and if the doctor has the slightest suspicion of MS—do a magnetic resonance (MR) scan. This test often reveals small abnormalities in the brain that help the doctor make the diagnosis of MS. If these abnormalities are common and occur in a specific, well-accepted pattern, the radiologist can strongly suggest the diagnosis of MS. When there are only a few tiny abnormalities with no specific localization, the doctor cannot make a definite diagnosis; but their presence should make the doctor aware of the strong possibility that the illness causing the fatigue is MS. Some time ago I performed a brain MR study in fifty-two CFS patients.[16] In nine patients, I found a small number of these tiny abnormalities. Despite the passage of time I was able to get back in touch with eight of these patients. The doctors of three of them had dropped the diagnosis of CFS. For two, the pattern of symptoms pointed to MS. These data indicate to me that patients with severe and chronic fatigue who have these "nonspecific" MR abnormalities may be in a different class from such patients without these abnormalities. It seems that some of them may actually have a mild form of MS.

Multiple sclerosis is well appreciated to be a severe, disabling, and often lethal disease. Like many other illnesses, it produces different degrees of severity from patient to patient. In some patients, fatigue and occasional neurological problems are the only complaints. For these individuals and for those with early MS, fatigue is a major complaint that is frequently ignored by the doctor. Thus, the diagnosis of MS or any of these other known causes of fatigue does not remove the need for the doctor to help the patient to deal with the problem. This sort of self-help will be the subject of later chapters of this book.

3 ❦ "Functional" Illnesses and Functional Causes of Fatigue

If 25 percent of patients visiting their doctor complain of severe and long-lasting fatigue, eliminating the illnesses discussed in the last chapter will still leave more than 5 percent whose complaints of fatigue cannot be explained. What is needed is consideration of a set of medical complaints that are called functional illnesses.

To understand the meaning of "functional" requires understanding of the medical word "syndrome." A syndrome is a collection of all that is known about a particular type of illness. Usually syndromes are built around illnesses that are poorly understood. Doctors recognize the existence of a syndrome if a group of sick patients look somewhat similar. Disease makes itself recognized by producing symptoms and signs. Symptoms are feelings such as nausea or pain that sick people report to their doctor. Signs, on the other hand, such as the elevated temperature indicative of fever or swollen lymph glands, are found by medical personnel while examining a sick person.

The Syndromic Approach
Gathering a set of signs and symptoms into a clinical disease entity or syndrome with a specific name allows medical progress to con-

tinue. The idea of the syndrome came from Thomas Sydenham, a seventeenth-century medical practitioner who revolutionized the history of medicine with his idea. What happened shortly after he popularized the concept of the syndrome is pretty much what happened in the mid-1980s with AIDS. A bright medical practitioner saw a group of patients who shared some signs and symptoms. The earliest reports were of a group of homosexual men who developed a rare form of cancer known as Kaposi's sarcoma and died of even rarer sorts of infectious disease, such as a type of tuberculosis that is seen in birds but only rarely in humans.

When an article about such an unusual syndrome appears in a medical journal with wide readership, doctors often write letters to the editor of the journal telling of their own experiences with similar cases. The combination of these anecdotes leads an individual who is focused on the "big picture" to put these individual stories together and to give the illness a name. When the seriousness and severity of AIDS were noted, the media labeled it the "gay plague."

The AIDS Example

The advantage of specifying a clinical disease entity is that researchers can investigate a group of patients who share similar signs and symptoms and use their similarities to try to find a biomedical marker of the disease. Again, that is what happened with AIDS. The first biomedical marker noted was that, as the disease progressed, the white blood cell (WBC) count decreased. White blood cells are important in protecting the body from infection, so a low WBC count was a clue to why the AIDS victim was catching such unusual infections. It pushed researchers to focus on the immune response of the AIDS victim. Soon they learned that one particular immune white blood cell—the CD3 or T cell—often fell to perilously low levels in an AIDS patient. When this happened, the AIDS victim fell prey to strange and extremely rare infectious diseases.

The discovery of this pathological disease entity allowed further refining of the concept of AIDS. This group of very similar patients was tested to see if some infectious agent had attacked their immune systems. As is now history, this idea proved to be a reality; the human immunodeficiency virus (HIV) was discovered, and a blood test for its presence was developed. Thus the clinical disease entity allowed researchers to assemble a group of patients who were so alike that the cause of the illness could be found. The process could then continue to its final step—use of the syndromic approach to test a specific drug or vaccination.

To finish the story of the syndromic approach, let me move to an illness caused by an infectious agent that is treatable—sore throat caused by the streptococcus bacteria. The miracle of the mid-twentieth century was the discovery of antibiotics. Even tiny doses of penicillin would cure a strep throat. Imagine the outcome if penicillin were given to one hundred consecutive patients with severe sore throat, fever, and swollen glands. Since the signs and symptoms I have just described constitute a syndrome, it can have many causes. These could include bacteria other than strep and many different viruses (including those that cause mononucleosis). Assume that the sore throat syndromes of twenty of these hundred patients were caused by strep. Curing twenty of one hundred patients would be impressive, but not front-page news. But imagine the excitement after doctors had learned how to identify the streptococcus bacteria as one of the causes of the sore throat syndrome. Developing the lab test meant that the doctor no longer had to rely solely on clinical judgment. Now she or he could swab the back of the throat and several days later learn that indeed the cause of the problem was strep. New techniques already in doctors' hands allow the diagnosis to be made in just a few hours.

Using this test, the doctor could identify all twenty patients with strep as the cause of their sore throat. Imagine the reaction when penicillin was given to that group of patients. A 100-percent cure rate!

Now *that* was front-page news. This story differs from the AIDS story in that medical science has not yet identified the antiviral agent that will kill or stop HIV. But it is obvious that this is coming. The news coming out of the summer 1996 AIDS meeting in Vancouver was that the number of viral particles—known as the viral burden—could be strikingly reduced by using a combination of available medicines. That certainly is the first step toward a cure. In fact, a recent report from the University of Minnesota suggests that thirty months of combined therapy can wipe out the virus from lymph nodes, which are its reservoir.[1]

In contrast to the AIDS story, many illnesses are still at the clinical disease entity level. We do not know what causes them, and we do not have a specific diagnostic test. For diseases in this category, it would be difficult to determine if any particular treatment was effective because the clinical disease entity may harbor diseases that look the same but have different causes.

Epilepsy vs. Pseudoepilepsy
An example of this comes from the discipline of neurology. A patient has a seizure in which he shakes all over and seems to lose contact with the world. The first thing the neurologist must determine is whether this is epilepsy, a disease of the brain, or a psychological aberration known as pseudoepilepsy manifesting itself as a pseudoseizure. In the past, two things allowed this determination: the pattern of the seizure, and whether it was accompanied by abnormal electrical activity in the brain as measured by an electroencephalograph (EEG). When the movements were repetitive and accompanied by loss of consciousness with loud deep breathing, epilepsy could be diagnosed whether or not the EEG was positive. Or when the movements were those thought not to reflect epilepsy—for instance, pelvic thrusts—the doctor was safe in making the diagnosis of epilepsy when the EEG was abnormal at the time the movements were taking place.

When the movements were not what the doctor expected, and the EEG was normal, the doctor was led to believe that the seizure was not caused by a problem in the brain but was instead a pseudoseizure. Imagine the consternation when that long-held belief fell. A report using newer EEG technology showed that such patients could have abnormal EEGs after all.[2]

Even when the diagnosis of epilepsy is made from an abnormal EEG, the cause may still be problematic. Most causes of epilepsy are unknown. Thus when the brain of such patients is examined, even at autopsy, abnormalities are only rarely found. The problem that causes this amazing change in behavior, which our language rightly terms a "seizure," has to be one that exists beneath the level that any microscope can detect. This level is the so-called functional level—where some sort of abnormality exists but cannot be seen or pinpointed.

In contrast, other forms of epilepsy have causes that can be seen. The most common is a brain tumor or a stroke that damages a part of the brain. Either results in irritation in a part of the brain that is manifested by the clinical syndrome known as a seizure.

"Functional" Illnesses

One definition of the word "functional," then, is a process that cannot be seen by current technology. A second definition is that the process is produced by emotional or nonorganic causes. Thus, some would call pseudoepilepsy a functional disorder. Again the history of medicine helps. Some functional illnesses—those that are thought not to be organic—turn out to be real medical illnesses but without a visible pathology. Besides epilepsy, common examples include depression, schizophrenia, and migraine. For many decades psychotherapy was the only treatment thought to be effective in disorders such as these. Over time, however, medical research has uncovered subtle abnormalities in brain function or anatomy for each of these illnesses. The indications are that each is a brain disease. When no such evidence exists, the syndrome is considered functional. The obvious lesson taught by the history of medicine is that many illnesses thought to be functional may need to be reclassified as organic, thanks to the development of new and improved diagnostic tools.

Let us now examine a group of functional illnesses that overlap. What they have in common is "fatigue plus." By that I mean that fatigue is but one of a number of symptoms constituting each of these functional illnesses. More important, since none of these illnesses has an effective biomedical diagnostic test or a known pathology, each can only be described as a clinical disease entity. The description of new clinical disease entities is, by definition, highly personalized. Medical investigators see best what they are trained to look for, and often overlook medical problems with which they do not feel very competent professionally. Thus, any one description of a clinical disease entity can overlap other descriptions made by physicians in different disciplines. This is to be expected before someone recognizes that these different "syndromes" are in fact variations of the same entity.

This seems to be the case with existing descriptions of conditions that can produce long-lived and severe fatigue: neurasthenia, the effort syndrome, hyperventilation, multiple chemical sensitivity, fibromyalgia, and the chronic fatigue syndrome. I will devote the remainder of this chapter and the next one to a description of each of these conditions and conclude with an evaluation of their similarities and differences (if any).

First I need to introduce one other concept, the notion of lumpers and splitters. Lumpers say, "Well, this illness looks a lot like this other one, so let's lump them together." Splitters, on the other hand, look for ways to split any one illness into subgroups. In order for the concept of the "syndrome" to allow us to distill a group of patients that all have the same medical problem, the splitters have to come out on top.

Neurasthenia

Now let's turn to those illnesses characterized by "fatigue plus." Historically, the place to start is with neurasthenia, first recognized in the nineteenth century.[3] The illness was principally characterized by the presence of profound fatiguability of body and mind—a slowing of normal mental abilities, accompanied by problems with attention and concentration. Myriad other symptoms were associated with this fatigue. The splitters divided neurasthenia into gastric, cardiac, or pulmonary subtypes, according to the organ producing the most symptoms in any particular patient. Neurasthenia was thought to be an organic brain disease and was found predominantly in the higher socioeconomic classes. When thirty to forty years of research had produced no biomedical marker or obvious cause of this syndrome, the idea arose that it was not a "real" illness but instead was a psychiatric problem related to hypochondriasis. Indeed, according to one formulation it was simply a type of depression. Because the symptoms of neurasthenia appeared to fit other psychiatric diagnoses, neurasthenia as a diagnosis started to disappear from Western medicine.

All the same, neurasthenia appears to be a popular diagnosis in China. Medical anthropologists attribute its frequency there as an indication that it is being diagnosed instead of depression, and that social factors within Chinese society lead to a diagnosis of neurasthenia before the diagnosis of depression is entertained.[4] Although neurasthenia has been subsumed by other psychiatric diagnoses in the United States, its existence in other parts of the world has led to its inclusion in an international classification of mental and behavioral disorders as one of a group of neurotic disorders. The term "neurotic" again suggests the word "functional"—that the problem is one of personality and character rather than an actual disease. The diagnosis demands either persistent and distressing complaints of increased fatigue after mental effort, or persistent and distressing complaints of bodily weakness and exhaustion after minimal effort. In addition, the patient must complain of at least two of the following: muscle aches or pains, dizziness, headache, sleep disturbance, inability to relax, irritability, and dyspepsia or indigestion. As we shall see, this diagnosis clearly overlaps with others described in this chapter. It is not known whether the current formulation, that this is a functional neurotic disorder or some more complicated organic disease, is correct.

The Effort Syndrome

Like neurasthenia, the effort syndrome was born in the nineteenth century.[5] It was initially reported in soldiers, who complained of severe exhaustion as well as shortness of breath and a rapid pulse following minimal effort. Subsequently the illness was recognized in civilians, affecting women twice as often as men and often occurring in successive generations of the same family. Symptoms included fatigue, breathlessness, sweats, the feeling of one's heart beating, dizziness, and chest pain. The resemblance of these symptoms to those produced by fear or anxiety caused several prominent cardiologists to label it an emotional disorder.

However, a host of studies suggest that the problem is not a mental one so much as a problem in the parts of the body that control the function of the heart, the blood vessels, and other organs. In general these organs are controlled by nerves, which make them operate faster or slower, and by hormones, which are substances in the blood that reach these organs via their blood supply to have similar effects on organ function. Because abnormalities in these "neurohormonal" systems have been found in these patients, one current idea is that the syndrome is not an emotional disorder so much as it is an abnormality in neurohormonal functioning and thus a physical illness.[6]

Mitral Valve Prolapse Syndrome

The effort syndrome really allowed the splitters to go to work. One group of these patients has been found to have a laboratory abnormality called mitral valve prolapse (MVP);[7] in fact, this is what most cardiologists think effort syndrome is. The mitral valve is the part of the heart that allows the principal pumping chamber, the left ventricle, to pump blood throughout the rest of the body. When the mitral valve does not function correctly and allows a backwash of blood, the affected person is at risk for serious heart problems.[8] What happens in these patients is that the valve is actually diseased and does not close properly or is a bit too big and floppy. In either case, the valve is pushed by the emerging blood and its leaflets prolapse into the neighboring cardiac compartment, the left atrium. If the fit of the prolapsed valve is not tight, blood backwashes into the atrium and the doctor can hear a murmur.

The majority of people with mitral valve prolapse do not have such a severe disorder, in that they do not experience this backward regurgitation of blood. Their valve does prolapse, but its edges are apposed tightly enough so that blood does not reflux into the left atrium. Many of these individuals—again usually women—have no symptoms at all and thus are unaware they have MVP. Since MVP is such a common laboratory abnormality in young women, it is not clear whether it is a marker for some other problem, an accidental occurrence, or somehow produces the many complaints expressed by some MVP patients. When one realizes that MVP becomes less common in older women, one begins to wonder just how important it actually is.

To complicate matters further, some people have the identical complaints of chest pain, palpitation, dizziness, and fatigue but have totally normal hearts. As in the patient with MVP, these symptoms may occur spontaneously or may follow effort. In both MVP patients and this group of patients, abnormalities of the systems controlling the heart have been found. These seem to differ from the abnormalities found in anxious people who have different symptoms from those in the effort syndrome group. Has following the splitters' path helped or hindered our understanding? What is clear is that a series of complaints related to the body's response to effort exist in a group of people—usually women. As we shall see, this syndromic pattern occurs over and over in illnesses that have other names. The idea that emerges is that these are all pieces of the same functional illness, which produces many different symptoms.

Hyperventilation

The story is very similar for hyperventilation.[9] In fact, one interpretation of the effort syndrome is that it is caused by hyperventilation.[10] Differences in classification arise because the chief complaints of people with hyperventilation are chest pain, shortness of breath, dizziness, faintness, and "air hunger" (the inability to take a satisfying breath). Fatigue, although always present, is a less dramatic component, so is often ignored by the doctor.

Hyperventilation means that a person breathes either faster or deeper than necessary. (This syndrome also is seen three times more often in women than men.)[11] You can detect hyperventilation in yourself if you breathe faster than eighteen times a minute, or if you sigh or yawn frequently while you breathe. There are two significant results of such hyperventilation or overbreathing. First, the person with the problem has to work more to breathe than a normal person, and this additional work can produce fatigue. Second, overbreathing changes blood chemistry in a way that produces symptoms. What happens is that the level of carbon dioxide in the blood decreases with overbreathing. This produces an almost immediate change in the blood's acid-base balance, which in turn produces symptoms such as feelings of numbness, dizziness, or faintness, and anxiety; a profound sense of fatigue usually accompanies these symptoms. Similarly, these changes in the blood's acid-base balance have additional consequences for organ function. By decreasing the flow of blood to an organ, symptoms such as pain can occur.

Although the clinical syndrome of hyperventilation has been recognized for decades, its cause remains questionable. As is so often the case with functional disorders, many physicians thought that it represented a bodily manifestation of an emotional disorder such as anxiety or nervousness. However, when groups of hyperventilators were given psychiatric evaluations, less than half fit this stereotype.[12] The response to therapy sometimes helps with the diagnosis. The symptoms related to low blood levels of carbon dioxide can be totally stopped by having the hyperventilating patient breathe into a closed bag held tight against the face; exhaled carbon dioxide does not escape to the open air but instead is trapped in the bag, where it is rebreathed. This treatment prevents the blood carbon dioxide level from falling. It is therefore an excellent way to diagnose the problem, and can be the way to treat it. This form of treatment can be of value for patients who have developed hyperventilation either as a bodily response to emotion or stress or even to those who have it as a bad habit—like thumb sucking or nail biting in an adult. So if you think you may be hyperventilating, try the paper bag test. Frequently, however, this type of rebreathing treatment is ineffective.

Surprisingly little attention has been paid to trying to understand the reason for hyperventilation in the majority of patients who do not have a psychiatric basis for their problem. Perhaps one reason is the underlying medical belief that this syndrome *must* have an emotional cause; but, as we shall see in a later chapter, the belief is more often wrong than right. An alternative is that the hyperventilator has a problem somewhat akin to that of the individual with fatigue and the sensation of palpitation: something is wrong in the brain's control of the internal organs—for the hyperventilator, the lungs; for the patient with palpitation and chest pain, the heart. Surprisingly, about a third of these patients turn out to have subtle but definite lung disease.[13] One of these lung problems might be mild asthma, which can often make breathing somewhat difficult and thus lead to overbreathing.

Evidence of lung disease was found only because the patients with hyperventilation were subjected to an intensive medical evaluation, one that would never have been done if it were not part of a scientific study. The fact that so many organic reasons for hyperventilation were found in this study should make any doctor cautious about attributing hyperventilation solely to emotional factors. This leap from belief to fact occurs all too often in medicine today.

Multiple Chemical Sensitivity
Another functional cause of fatigue is an illness known as multiple chemical sensitivity (MCS), which is just beginning to wend its way through the syndromic approach. At first, it was described by a number of doctors in a broad clinical way. Basically the problem is one of symptoms following exposure to some chemical or toxin. What often happens is that an individual reports being very sensitive to almost any odor following the original chemical exposure. It is as if the original exposure changes the person's sensitivity to strong odorants and the individual seems to become extremely reactive to almost any smell. Thus the illness might have begun after having the rugs cleaned in one's home, or after starting a job in a newly constructed building. Symptoms might include severe fatigue, pain, difficulty in concentrating, and abdominal and bowel problems. The fact that such symptoms follow exposure to certain odorants commonly leads the affected person to try to avoid them. If the problem is relatively minor, this is not too difficult. Patients can avoid walking down the aisle in the supermarket where detergents are found. But sometimes it is harder to avoid aromas; cigarette smoke and perfumes are frequent culprits. Because affected individuals feel better when they avoid such odors, they may make major life changes to achieve this goal. I have seen patients wear ventilators like those used by coal miners or move to remote parts of the country where contact with others is minimal.
    Recently a large group of doctors was polled in an effort to deter-

mine what criteria are necessary to make the diagnosis of MCS.[14] The problem with this approach is that it is the doctors who are deciding what the illness is, and it is possible that they may not know the complete pattern of symptoms. A consensus approach is useful but obviously it depends on who is polled. If all the doctors have the same background, they will focus on problems that are both familiar and interesting. In contrast, the patient may have problems that have never been verbalized because the doctor did not think to inquire about them. This problem in communication between patient and physician is one that I will discuss in Chapter 5.

In fact, this was the synopsis with MCS. Because the doctors who were initially interested in this disorder were often allergists or physicians in occupational or job-related medicine, the diagnosis of MCS was tied heavily to exposure to chemicals, production of symptoms upon exposure to the same chemicals, and reduction of symptoms when exposure was reduced. Probably owing to this same skew, the illness has been also labeled the total allergy syndrome or the environmental illness.[15]

Surprisingly, thousands of Persian Gulf veterans returned from that war with many of the complaints enumerated in the above syndromes; these include fatigue, achiness, headache, sensitivity to chemicals, and abdominal distress. Following previous military actions these complaints may have been ignored as medically trivial or considered to be either malingering or some minor emotional problem. After the Persian Gulf, the Department of Veterans Affairs took the problem seriously and encouraged medical scientists to research the problem.

Because of our interest in the medical causes of fatigue, my colleagues and I responded to this challenge by sending a questionnaire to a group of veterans who, following their tour of duty in the Gulf, had gone to a Veterans Administration (VA) hospital for a physical examination. A previous evaluation had found that about 15 percent of these veterans had no medical complaints, whereas the remaining 85 percent had symptoms and felt ill. The questionnaire was essentially the one we had developed to evaluate people for the existence of chronic fatigue syndrome. We also asked veterans whether they thought they were especially sensitive to certain chemicals and whether they had been forced to change their usual style of living because of chemical or food sensitivity. If a veteran answered affirmatively to both of these questions, we labeled him as chemically sensitive. We asked whether he was suffering from fatigue, and if so, we inquired about its duration and its effect on his normal degree of activity. (I use the masculine pronoun here because, in contrast to the civilian disorders discussed earlier in this chapter, the fatiguing illness in the Gulf veteran follows the demographics of military personnel in being predominantly a disorder of men. Female veterans were in the minority, yet it may be important to note that more of them were in the patient group than would have been predicted based on their numbers in the Gulf.)

The results were surprising. Over 60 percent of the veterans responding to our questionnaire indicated that they were suffering from fatigue lasting more than six months. And the responses of 6 percent were consistent with the diagnosis of CFS. This is a much higher proportion than the 0.3 percent maximal rate found in one thousand consecutive patients in general medical practice.[16] Obviously, the difference is that we relied solely on the answers to our questionnaire, whereas the other study performed thorough medical evaluations. So our 6 percent figure is probably artificially high. Still, it is very impressive and suggests that something about the veterans' experience in the Persian Gulf triggered a mini-epidemic of CFS.

Of equal importance was our finding that vets with chronic fatigue syndrome often also had MCS. This suggests that the two diagnoses overlap. We are checking this possibility in nonveteran patients with CFS. A preliminary appraisal by a group in Seattle found little difference between CFS and MCS patients.[17] If this observation can be confirmed, we will need to look at chemical exposure as a possible cause of severe fatiguing illness. But if the nonveterans with chronic fatigue syndrome do not have a frequent problem with multiple chemical sensitivity while veterans with CFS do, this will suggest that the CFS in the veterans has a different cause—possibly related to chemical exposure—than that in the nonveterans.

Somatization Disorder and Hysteria

The final diagnostic group to be reviewed in this chapter is patients with somatization disorder,[18] a psychiatric diagnosis in the family of hypochondriasis. Once more, this diagnosis is much more frequent in women than in men. Patients are diagnosed as having somatization disorder if their diverse medical complaints are not thought by competent medical personnel to have a medical cause. Thus, somatization is thought to be either an emotional disorder or a hypersensitivity to one's bodily sensations. Sexual abuse or physical illness before the age of eighteen[19] seem to be factors that can lead to somatization. It is well known that people with somatization disorder overutilize medical resources.[20] Furthermore, their bodily concerns can lead to treatments—even surgery—that might not be reliably indicated. However, the concept that patients with multiple medical complaints of no known cause must have a psychiatric disorder certainly goes against the grain of medical history, as we have already seen.

An advanced form of somatization called hysteria provides an example.[21] In somatization, patients have symptoms—that is, medical complaints—that cannot be explained. In hysteria, patients have signs—abnormalities that the doctor finds on examination—that cannot be explained. These can be as dramatic as seizures or paralyses. E. T. O. Slater, with his coworkers, made an important study of a group of hysterics.[22] Following them over a five-year period, he found that 25 percent of these individuals, who were thought to have a mental illness, actually were harboring a physical disease that almost certainly was responsible for their symptoms and signs. Although the majority of the hysterics followed probably did have a psychiatric disorder, an appreciable minority had an illness that their doctors were unable to diagnose when symptoms, and even signs, of the disease developed. The conclusion derived from this study can be extended to patients who receive a new diagnosis of somatization disorder or hysteria—especially those who develop these symptoms suddenly with no prior history: some of you will have organic illnesses that cannot be identified with 100 percent surety today.

Somatization—the tendency to amplify and focus on symptoms—does exist and does cause the somatizing individual to consume large and unnecessary amounts of medical care. The task of the researcher is to come up with a formula to determine who has the hypochondriacal tendency and who is in the early stages of an as-yet undiagnosed disease.

4 (Chronic Fatigue Syndrome

In the last chapter we talked about illnesses in which the significance of chronic fatigue has tended to be overlooked. For instance, whereas fatigue is known to be a symptom of mitral valve prolapse, it is not considered an important problem, and the severity and frequency of fatigue in MVP have not been studied.

But there are two other, rather common illnesses where chronic— severe and long-lasting—fatigue is the major focus of interest. In chronic fatigue syndrome and fibromyalgia, severe fatigue is a principal component of the clinical presentation. Again, the descriptions of these diseases were very much influenced by the backgrounds of the physicians who initially noticed them.

Fibromyalgia (FM) provides the telling example. It is an illness characterized by fatigue, diffuse pain and/or stiffness, and tenderness that is often striking at certain points of the body. The diagnostic criteria for FM are as follows:[1]

1. Pain is considered widespread when *all of the following are present:* pain in the left side of the body, pain in the right side of the body, pain above the waist, and pain below the waist.

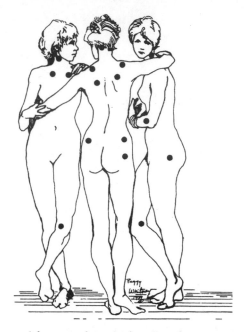

Figure 1 There are eighteen tender point locations that are pressed with the thumb at 9 pounds of force to make the diagnosis of fibromyalgia. Sixteen tender points have been superimposed on Regnault's 1793 painting of *The Three Graces;* not shown are the points on the right side of the nape of the neck and the right elbow. Courtesy of Dr. Fred Wolfe.

In addition, pain must exist in either the neck, the low back, or along the spine or over the chest. Shoulder or buttock pain on one side counts toward pain on that side of the body; "low back" pain counts as pain below the waist.

2. When pressure of about 9 pounds is applied to each point shown in Figure 1, the tender point criterion is met if pain is reported in at least eleven sites.

To make the diagnosis, doctors press at each of the eighteen points shown; if patients report pain at eleven or more of these sites as well as widespread spontaneous pain, they receive the diagnosis of

FM. This simplified way of making a diagnosis focuses on pain and ignores other symptoms such as fatigue, even though they may be prominent.

Because the pain of FM was most often seen in muscles and joints, individuals with this problem would often wind up in the offices of rheumatologists, who focus mostly on joint and muscle problems. However, patients with fibromyalgia have been reevaluated with the realization that FM is an illness where severe and chronic fatigue is a major problem.[2] Although fibromyalgia can occur without fatigue, when fatigue is a prominent component, fibromyalgia is identical to the illness one usually thinks of when speaking of severe and chronic fatigue—chronic fatigue syndrome, or CFS.

The History and Definition of CFS

Chronic fatigue syndrome became a focus of medical attention because of reports of what appeared to be epidemics of a polio-like infection, which clearly differed from polio in that the muscles in the affected patients never lost their bulk and never became paralyzed. Reports of such epidemics appeared as early as 1934. Several outbreaks in the 1950s in London attracted the attention of a physician who was expert in infectious diseases. Dr. Melvin Ramsay is probably most responsible for the illness' remaining in the public eye. In one such mini-epidemic, or cluster of cases, in a London hospital, he noted the similarity between the complaints of the affected employees and those of patients whose illness did not begin in such a cluster; the medical term for illness onset that does not appear in a cluster or epidemic form is "endemic" or "sporadic." Ramsay became so fascinated with the illness that he spent much of his professional life studying it and caring for patients with the problem.[3]

Probably because no physician with Dr. Ramsay's interest in this illness was living in North America, an important 1959 review of past epidemics of severe fatiguing illness in the American medical literature[4] was forgotten until late 1984. At that time an epidemic of such an illness in Incline Village, Nevada, attracted the attention of the medical community.[5] This mini-epidemic prompted physicians around the world to start paying attention to this medical problem. That focus of attention is evident by the wealth of medical commentaries on the illness from many countries and in many different languages.[6]

The illness that occurred in the small Nevada village resembled acute infectious mononucleosis (mono) in that symptoms included sudden onset, a feeling of weakness, fatigue, fever, sore throat, swollen glands, achiness, difficulty with sleep, and problems of attention and concentration. Unlike mono, which in the great majority of cases disappears after weeks or several months, many of the Nevada patients continued to complain of symptoms for six months or more. Because of the similarity, the illness soon was named chronic mononucleosis. As in the previously reported mini-epidemics, most patients recovered; but some remained sick for many months or even years afterward.

Early Theories

Because the illness was thought to be a chronic form of mono, attention was drawn to the virus known to cause that illness—the Epstein-Barr virus (EBV). The state of knowledge about this virus in 1985 was that after infection, the virus did not disappear from the system like other viruses that produced the flu. Instead, it went into hiding or, to use the medical term, became latent. EBV is one member of the class of viruses known as herpesviruses. The best-known example is herpesvirus-1, the virus that produces cold sores or fever sores in people. It produces an initial illness resembling the flu, after which the virus goes into hiding in the nerve that carries sensation from the lip to the brain. Thereafter the virus does not cause a flu-like syndrome again, but instead produces the very common fever sore. Following some stress—be it fever or exposure to bright sunlight—the virus comes out of hiding, travels down the nerve to the lip, where it does its usual damage, nearly always in exactly the same spot.

This pattern of going latent and then reactivating also occurs for the Epstein-Barr virus, but reactivation of the EBV infection is much less common than is true of fever sores. Reactivation can occur in patients with diseases such as AIDS, which interfere with the immune system's ability to repulse viral challenges. When there is immune dysfunction, the reactivated viral illness is usually much more serious than the usual case of mono and can even be lethal. Because of medical reports tying EBV infection to prolonged fatiguing illness, it was natural to assume that "chronic mononucleosis" was in fact "chronic EBV infection." This idea was helped along by finding abnormal EBV blood tests in chronically fatigued patients.[7]

Unfortunately, as is so often true in medicine, what makes sense and what is true are not always the same. The original thinking was that these abnormal EBV blood tests indicated that the virus was active in the body and thus responsible for the patients' medical complaints. But reports appeared indicating that people who had returned to normal health after mono, as well as those with no history of mono, could have the same "abnormal" EBV blood tests.[8] Finding supposedly abnormal laboratory results in healthy people meant that the test results really were not abnormal. Therefore, the doctor could not use abnormal EBV blood tests to help with diagnosis. The idea that EBV was the cause of chronic fatiguing illness—even that following an infection that looked like infectious mononucleosis—quickly fell out of favor.

The Name and the Appearance of CFS
Because the cause of this strange lingering illness was not as clear as was initially thought, physicians and medical scientists reverted to using the "syndromic" approach. Their first step was to come up with a name for the illness. "Chronic EBV infection" obviously was no

longer suitable. The British had called the epidemic presentation of this illness myalgic encephalomyelitis (ME), and the term soon was applied to patients with chronic fatigue whose illness did not begin in an epidemic. Although "ME" remains in use in much of the United Kingdom, many researchers had trouble with the name because the word "encephalomyelitis" indicates a definite pathological infectious-type abnormality in the brain and spinal cord, and no one has found such an abnormality. Calling the illness "chronic fatigue syndrome," or CFS, seemed a reasonable alternative—at least until some definitive cause was found. Essentially, the illness was defined as new onset of persistent or recurring fatigue, lasting at least six months and having no known medical cause—plus.

The "plus" includes the presence of a number of symptoms including headache, weakness, muscle pain, joint pain, difficulty with sleep (either insomnia, sleeping too much, or lacking restful sleep), difficulty with concentration, attention or memory, feverishness, sore throat, painful lymph glands, and a worsening of fatigue after relatively mild physical exertion. Until very recently, no worldwide agreement existed on how to evaluate these symptoms to arrive at a diagnosis. From 1988 to 1991, committees of experts in several countries established different but overlapping case definitions of CFS. The term "case definition" means a set of criteria, agreed on by a consensus of experts, that define a specific clinical syndrome. The case definition of CFS in the United States, published in 1988 and modified several years later,[9] allowed the diagnosis if the fatigue was so severe as to reduce activity by at least 50 percent, lasted at least six months, and was accompanied by at least eight of the above symptoms (see Table 2). In Great Britain, the fatigue had to be present for at least half the six-month minimum and had to be severe, disabling, and affect physical and mental functioning. In Australia, the fatigue had to disrupt daily activities, and the patient had to complain of postexertional fatigue and a new problem with concentration or short-term memory.

Table 2 U.S. Case Definition of Chronic Fatigue Syndrome, 1988

Major Criteria:

1. Persisting or relapsing fatigue or easy fatigability that does not involve bedrest and is severe enough to reduce daily activity by at least 50 percent
2. Other chronic clinical conditions have been excluded, including preexisting psychiatric diseases

Minor Criteria:
Report of persistent or recurring symptoms lasting at least six months.
1. Mild fever (99.5° to 101.5° oral) or chills
2. Sore throat
3. Painful lymph nodes in front or back of the neck or under the arms
4. Unexplained generalized muscle weakness
5. Muscle discomfort or myalgia
6. Prolonged (more than twenty-four hours) generalized fatigue following previously tolerable levels of exercise
7. New, generalized headaches
8. Pain in more than one joint without redness or swelling
9. Neuropsychological symptoms (one or more of following)
   a. Photophobia
   b. Brief duration patches of blindness (i.e., visual scotomata)
   c. Forgetfulness
   d. Excessive irritability
   e. Confusion
   f. Difficulty in thinking
   g. Inability to concentrate
   h. Depression (following illness onset)
10. Sleep disturbance (hypersomnia or insomnia)
11. Illness onset occurring over hours to a few days (sudden onset)

Diagnosis requires both major criteria and at least eight of the minor criteria.

Sources: G. P. Holmes, J. E. Kaplan, N. M. Gantz, et al., "Chronic Fatigue Syndrome: A Working Case Definition," *Annals of Internal Medicine* 108 (1988): 387–389.

The problem with any such consensus-type definition is that it is based on opinion and impression rather than fact. This is especially true when a medical condition is first being recognized, as is currently the case with multiple chemical sensitivity. As facts accumulate, the clinical case definition must change to accommodate new knowledge. This process of sculpting the definition continues until a biomedical marker is found; then diagnosis is based on a combination of the clinical and the pathological findings. In addition, the case definition can itself change if problems are perceived to exist.

The 1994 International Case Definition
The existence of three somewhat different case definitions was an immediate concern. Would advances based on patients diagnosed with the Australian case definition hold if applied to patients diagnosed with one of the other case definitions? Obviously a uniform worldwide case definition would obviate this problem. Another concern focused on chronically fatigued patients whose illness did not fulfill any of the three case definitions. What about, for example, an American patient with six months of severe fatigue who had only six or seven of the original list of eleven accompanying symptoms? Was this patient somehow different from the patient who had eight symptoms on the list and thus could receive the diagnosis of CFS?[10] The concern here was that strict application of the available case definitions excluded patients from receiving the diagnosis of CFS for no rational reason. If there was no important difference between these two patient examples, then it made sense to give both patients the diagnosis of chronic fatigue syndrome. In addition, the idea of requiring fewer symptoms to fulfill a revised case definition of CFS was attractive to several groups of experts who had shown that patients with many bodily complaints tend to have far more psychiatric problems (and perhaps a psychiatric cause for their complaints) than do CFS patients with fewer complaints.[11] The reasoning was that by requiring fewer complaints to receive the diagnosis of CFS, these patients might increase the size of the group with no psychiatric cause of their chronic fatigue.

To deal with these concerns and to try to get consensus across national borders, an international group of physicians of which I was part who are acknowledged experts in CFS reconsidered the original case definition and in 1994 made available a changed

Table 3 International Case Definition of Chronic Fatigue Syndrome, 1994

Medically unexplained, persistent, or relapsing chronic fatigue that is of new or definite onset
   Not due to exertion, not relieved by rest
   Results in substantial reduction in previous levels of occupational, educational, social, or personal activities
Concurrent occurrence of four or more of the following symptoms
   Must have persisted or recurred for six or more consecutive months of illness
   Must not have predated fatigue
   Impairment in short-term memory or concentration severe enough to cause substantial reduction in previous levels of occupational, educational, social, or personal activities
   Painful lymph nodes in front or back of the neck or under the arms
   Sore throat
   Muscle pain
   Pain in more than one joint without redness or swelling
   Headaches of a new type
   Unrefreshing sleep
   Postexertional malaise lasting more than twenty-four hours

Source: K. Fukuda, S. E. Straus, I. Hickie, et al., "The Chronic Fatigue Syndrome: A Comprehensive Approach to Its Definition and Study," *Annals of Internal Medicine* 121 (1994): 953–959.

version (see Table 3).[12] Our group reasoned that it would be advisable to give larger numbers of patients the diagnosis of CFS and sort out any differences later. To do this, the panel replaced the 50 percent reduction in activity requirement with the requirement that the fatigue had to produce a substantial decrease in school, work, social, or personal activities. It also dropped some of the symptoms that were hard to substantiate, such as feverishness and weakness. The new list included headache, sore throat, painful lymph glands, muscle pain, joint pain, unrefreshing sleep, postexertional malaise, and problems with short-term memory or concentration that were severe enough to produce a substantial decrease in activity. And now the case definition required problems with only four of these symptoms over the six-month period for a patient to receive the diagnosis of CFS. That diagnosis is not made in patients who

Fatigue

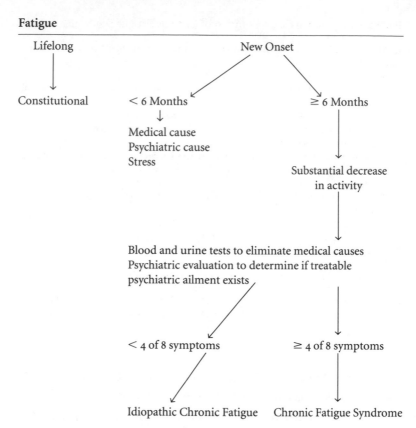

Figure 2 Flow chart for the diagnosis of chronic fatigue syndrome in accordance with the 1994 case definition.

have experienced schizophrenia, manic-depressive illness, bulimia, or substance abuse. Figure 2 shows how a doctor would arrive at the CFS diagnosis.

An obvious consequence of relaxing the requirements is that many more patients will receive the diagnosis of CFS. An additional group of patients with previously unexplained illness will now have an illness with a name. Even the vague name CFS is often very comforting to those who do not know why they feel ill. And having a diagnosis allows the severely affected CFS patient, disabled from the illness and unable to work, to try for financial help in the form of disability payments—either from his or her own insurance plan or from social security.

Grappling with the Case Definition

We now have a new case definition for CFS that will increase the number of people who receive the diagnosis. In thinking about this change, I reasoned that perhaps the greater pool of CFS patients would provide a broader range of severity of illness. For example, someone with severe fatigue but only four of the ancillary symptoms in the 1994 case definition would probably be less sick than another patient who had all eleven of the ancillary symptoms from the 1988 case definition. If I could identify two such groups of CFS patients, then I could test one of the reasons for developing the 1994 case definition—that there was no difference between patients who did not fulfill the original 1988 case definition and those who did. To define those groups, I had to grapple with the case definition, which posed one major problem for me. It said that all the symptoms could be "recurring"—that they could come and go. Under this definition a patient with serious problems lasting more than six months could come to my office feeling well on the day of that visit. Because I was concerned that it might be harder to find a cause for the illness in such a patient, I decided to modify the case definition to comprise two groups of CFS patients—those with "mild CFS" and those with "severe CFS."

To do this, I asked patients to rank the severity of their symptoms in the month prior to their office visit on a scale of 0 to 5: 0 represented no problem; 1, a mild problem; 2, a moderate problem; 3, a substantial problem; 4, a severe problem; and 5, a very severe problem. I defined a patient with "severe CFS" as one who fulfilled the original U.S. 1988 case definition but who also ranked the severity of symptoms in the month prior to the office visit at 3 or higher on the above scale.

I then defined a patient with "mild CFS" using the same severity criteria of 3 or higher but requiring only four to six symptoms in the month prior to the office visit. My working hypothesis was that by virtue of having fewer symptoms, this group was probably not as sick as the "severe" group. A comparison of the two groups showed one major difference, in how often patients complained of infectious-type symptoms: feverishness, chills, sore throat, or tender glands in the neck or under the arms. Seventy-six percent of the severe group reported having substantial problems with at least three of these symptoms in comparison to only 48 percent of the mild group. This observation indicates that the pattern of CFS symptoms for the mild group differs from that of the severe group. It is not just that there are fewer symptoms overall, but that the presence of certain symptoms—specifically the infectious-type ones—is less frequent and/or less intense.

This finding has several possible meanings. It certainly does not support the idea that one CFS patient is the "same" as the next in terms of the nature of their complaints. As I will soon explain, one explanation for the cause of CFS is that it is a long-term viral infection. However, if that were the case, one would logically expect infectious-type symptoms. Since these are much less common in the mild CFS group, an infectious cause is less likely for their illness. Furthermore, looking for an infectious cause in a combined group of mild and severe CFS patients would defeat the syndromic approach. If an infectious cause does in fact exist, mixing in patients with no apparent infection will make the agent even harder to find.

Symptom Amplifiers

This study did support my idea that there is a spectrum of severity of CFS—from mild to severe. We now know that certain conditions magnify symptom severity in CFS. Thus, having CFS plus one of these symptom amplifiers could convert mild CFS to severe CFS. One of these amplifiers relates to menstrual status of some women. Nearly every woman who ovulates experiences changes (food craving, bloating, or breast tenderness) that indicate an impending menstrual period. For as much as 7 percent of the female population, premenstrual symptoms are so severe that they require a physician's care. The symptoms of this premenstrual syndrome (PMS) include fatigue, difficulty concentrating and sleeping, headache, joint or muscle pain; so they overlap greatly with those seen in CFS.

It is conceivable that some women whose PMS produced "substantial" fatigue recurring for longer than six months might actually fulfill the relaxed 1994 case definition of CFS. Regardless of this possibility, what is clear is that when CFS and PMS occur at the same time, the symptoms of CFS become much worse premenstrually. One wonders whether PMS is a risk factor for later developing CFS.

Another major amplifier is the coexistence of fibromyalgia.[13] Dedra Buchwald, an internist at the University of Washington in Seattle, has compared her findings in CFS patients without fibromyalgia to a group who also fulfilled the case definition for FM (CFS/FM). Although both groups manifested the same symptoms, Dr. Buchwald found tender or enlarged lymph glands in the neck or under the arms more often in the CFS/FM group than in the group with just CFS. Moreover, she found that patients in the CFS/FM group were more disabled by their illness than those in the CFS-alone group.

Although some CFS patients have no problem continuing an active, albeit reduced, lifestyle, many CFS patients cannot do this and become fully disabled. Our Chronic Fatigue Syndrome Center in New Jersey has assessed the degree of disability among CFS patients, depressives, and patients with mild multiple sclerosis.[14] Fatigue is often a major complaint for patients with both depression and MS. But the level of disability for the depressed and MS patients was substantially less than for CFS patients.

In contrast to MS and depressed patients, CFS patients had substantial problems with the basic and intermediate activities of daily living (ADLs). Basic activities include self-care, moving in and out of bed or chair, and walking indoors. While ratings of these were nearly always in the normal range for patients with depression and mild MS, the majority of CFS patients reported significant problems with basic ADLs. The story was similar for intermediate ADLs. These include doing housework and errands, walking several blocks, climbing a flight of stairs, driving a car or using public transportation, and participating in vigorous activities such as strenuous sports. Patients with depression and mild MS usually reported no problems with these activities, while CFS patients were frequently at the dysfunctional level. Looked at another way, only 45 percent of the thirty-four CFS patients in one of our studies were able to work in contrast to 94 percent of mild MS patients and 82 percent of depressed patients. Implicit in these statistics is an element of social isolation and significantly impaired quality of life.[15]

The Prognosis in CFS
Our center studies CFS patients whose illness has not been of very long duration. So an important issue is to determine the long-term consequences of being diagnosed with CFS. We found that only 5 percent (two of our thirty-four patients) had returned to a normal life within two years of the time they participated in our studies. The majority of the remaining patients showed some, but not much, improvement. Another follow-up study was done by an Australian group three years after an initial evaluation.[16] The Australian case definition for CFS resembles the 1994 international case definition in that it is more liberal than the original 1988 American one. The 103 patients reevaluated had been sick for more than nine years on average. Five percent reported that they were back to normal. While nearly two-thirds of the patients noted improvement, almost half

were still unable to do any kind of work. These studies highlight the point that improvement is the rule, and complete recovery can occur. However, the road to recovery for many CFS patients is a long one and influenced by their coping style. Attempting to maintain improvement is associated with a better outcome, while focusing on symptoms and accommodating to the illness lead to further impairment.[17]

Researchers from London, Nijmegen (Holland), Baltimore, and Seattle have tried to identify factors that predict a successful or poor outcome from CFS.[18] In general, these studies indicate that younger patients, sick for a relatively short time, who have never had dysthymia or depression, will have the best outcomes. Also, CFS patients who do not attribute their illness solely to physical factors such as viral infection seem to have a greater chance of recovery.

Additional research suggests that patients' beliefs about the cause of their illness do not always relate to recovery. The relation is there for CFS patients who end up in a university CFS center after many physician visits. A London study showed that most of these patients attributed their illness to ME or to postviral fatigue syndrome.[19] In contrast, CFS patients who remain under the care of their general practitioner, and who have the same symptoms and disabilities as the patients at a major center, attributed their illness to psychological or psychosocial factors. Since illness outcome appears no different for the two groups, attribution may not be an important predictor of outcome; it may go hand in hand with longer duration and more severe illness, which ultimately bring the patient to a CFS specialist.

A Worldwide Problem, Predominantly of Women

The next question pertains to who gets CFS. The original focus was on adults, but children and adolescents are also stricken.[20] In addition to a large number of reports from the United States and the United Kingdom, others from Holland, Italy, and Germany indicate that the disease appears predominantly in women.[21] However, a Japanese study reports the same illness rate in men and women.[22] This finding raises the interesting possibility that CFS in Japan is a different illness, with perhaps different causes, from that seen in European countries. Nonetheless, the fact that medical journals from many different countries have published papers on CFS indicates that it is a worldwide problem.

The demographic data on our own "severe" CFS patients show that about 85 percent of our patients are women, and all but one of our eighty-seven patients are Caucasian and on the average well educated. Although the illness was originally labeled "yuppie flu" because of its apparent targeting of upper-middle-class women, our analysis of socioeconomic status in our patients indicates that the illness can affect people in all walks of life.

Based on efforts to identify CFS in minority populations in the United States, the disease seems unusual in people of African descent. There is a strong possibility that this racial disparity represents cultural differences concerning what constitutes illness among people of different backgrounds. Sociologists have identified striking differences among races and nationalities in such beliefs. Should a fatigued person of African descent not identify her fatigue as a problem, or not believe that her doctor would recognize it as such, she might not mention it. For a study to determine definitively which races are susceptible or resistant to CFS, epidemiologists (the scientists who study these issues) will have to circumvent these probable biases. One possible technique might be to telephone families on a random basis and ask the person who answers the phone if fatigue is a major problem for anyone living at that address. If the answer is affirmative, then a more complete assessment for CFS could be undertaken. Federal funds are currently supporting exactly this kind of study in an area of Chicago populated by people of diverse backgrounds and races.

Who Is at Risk?

Who is at risk of coming down with CFS? To determine risk, clinical epidemiologists ask a host of questions to a group of patients and to a comparison group of well people. This is called a case control study. Certainly if enough questions are asked, some differences between patients and controls may be due to chance alone. So any study assigning risk to a single factor requires follow-up studies for confirmation. Here is an example from my own work. In association with Dr. James Dobbins of the Centers for Disease Control (CDC), the principal U.S. government institution for medical epidemiology, we mailed questionnaires on a large number of possible risk factors to patients from my private practice and to healthy people whom we recruited from the university at which I work. The one factor that stood out in the patient group was exposure to various stressful events prior to the onset of illness; this was not a common occurrence in the healthy group.[23] We know that stress has major effects on resistance to viruses and on immune function, so this was exciting news indeed. Perhaps exposure to stressful events was the trigger for CFS.

We designed a follow-up study to test this finding. This time we used our center patients with severe CFS, and healthy controls whom we had identified by random digit dialing (a computer comes up with a list of random numbers within an area code, then recruiters call those numbers in an effort to get volunteers to serve as controls for an epidemiologic study). The results did not confirm the stress connection. That is, exposures to stress prior to CFS occurred at the same rate in the patients as during the same time period in the controls. Why the discrepancy?

The original study had used private patients who had not had the extensive evaluation of the patients at the research center, and case controls from my laboratory and from neighboring offices in the university. For the follow-up study, the patient group was more rigorously defined and the controls were people found at random—not all in the same general line of work and with the same interests. Finding healthy control subjects on a nonrandom basis could produce bias in the results, a possible explanation for the differences in the two studies. The value of techniques like random digit dialing to identify case controls becomes apparent.

The results in the two studies point to a basic scientific truth: "facts" change with additional research. A scientific result must stand the test of time, which requires that others are able to obtain—replicate—the same results. Even though the results of any one study may be stimulating and appear in the newspaper, they only really count when other groups find the same results as well.

With this background we can now turn to the few other case control epidemiological studies of risk in CFS. A study of seven children with CFS pointed toward recent ingestion of raw milk, similar symptoms in family members, and a history of allergy or asthma.[24] A later study from the CDC also found a tendency toward more allergies in the CFS group as well as an increased rate of chronic fatiguing illness in family members, but it could not confirm the relation with ingestion of raw milk.[25] A 1996 study could not confirm the allergy connection but did find that patients had exercised more regularly before onset of illness than controls.[26] This series of studies shows how the scientific process weeds out risk factors that are relatively weak. No major risk factor for CFS was identified, suggesting that more work must be done.

Is CFS a Form of Depression?

Medical explanations of CFS begin with depression. Today depression is no longer thought to be a functional illness that stems from environmental and emotional problems. Instead, genetic studies and drug trials indicate that it is a biological disorder of neurotransmitter physiology. Neurotransmitters are chemicals that connect one neuron to the next in the chain that controls the movement from thought to action. Here the illness resembles hypertension more than it does cancer. By this I mean that depression and hypertension are probably extremes of normal human behavior and/or experience, whereas cancer is never normal. One of the findings in depression is decreased amounts of certain brain neurotransmitters; these abnormalities are actually thought to cause the illness. When medicines are given that restore the appropriate levels of these neurotransmitters, the depression disappears and the patient can return to a normal life.

It is apparent that many of the symptoms of CFS overlap those of depression; the only symptoms of CFS that are not found in depression are the infectious symptoms of feverishness, sore throat, and swollen and tender glands. All the other symptoms—pain, confusion, weakness, sleep disorder—can be seen in depressed people. This finding has led some to believe that CFS is a form of depression.[27] One thing is clear: the majority of cases of moderate to severe, long-lasting fatigue report problems with life stress or anxiety.[28] However, these are individuals with fatigue but not CFS. Can we extrapolate the results of studies based on fatigued but otherwise healthy people to patients with CFS?

There is no totally definitive answer to this question. The problem is that it actually comprises several questions. One is whether prior serious psychiatric problems increase a person's risk of developing a chronic fatiguing illness. The answer seems to be, overwhelmingly, yes. If one looks at all CFS patients, a surprisingly large number had a serious problem with anxiety or depression before their CFS began.[29]

Working with a mixed (heterogeneous) group of patients whose illness has many different causes makes it difficult, if not impossible, to isolate and identify any one specific cause of the malady. An obvious tactic is to reduce this heterogeneity. Our center separates CFS patients with prior psychiatric diagnosis from those with no such history. It will be important to compare these two groups of patients to determine if prior psychiatric illness makes a CFS patient different from one who has never had psychiatric problems. In one such study we did not find any differences in immune tests of the two groups, but we did find that fewer of the prior psychiatric group were able to work than patients in the other group.[30] We interpret these results as predicting that the prognosis for recovery for this group may be less favorable than for the group with no prior psychiatric problems. Based on the immunological test results, CFS may be the same regardless of the patient's prior psychiatric history. It will be important to see whether this result holds for other biological variables, too.

The next issue has to do with the presence of psychiatric difficulties that started at the same time or after the CFS. If such a patient had a psychiatric problem *before* the onset of her illness, she might be in a different causal category than a patient who was previously well and then developed CFS and a psychiatric problem. It is possible that the first patient's CFS is a variant of her psychiatric problem, while the second patient may have developed the psychiatric problem because of the difficulties of having a chronic illness. So the reports of CFS patients having a high rate of psychiatric problems are not actually helpful, because they do not identify the number of patients for whom these problems are a new occurrence. The lack of such information makes it hard to decide on the importance of psychiatric factors in the genesis of CFS.

Our center has been rigorous in trying to define CFS in a way that will improve the consistency of the diagnosis from patient to patient. The goal again is to reduce heterogeneity. We used the severity criteria mentioned earlier. In a second modification of the original 1988 case definition, we excluded from the research any patient who had had a psychiatric diagnosis in the five years prior to the start of CFS. These modifications yielded a group of patients who were very symptomatic at the time of initial evaluation and who had no major psychiatric problems prior to the onset of chronic fatigue syndrome.

Of eighty-seven patients with severe CFS, by our modified case definition, psychiatric testing revealed that thirty-three had a psychiatric illness that had begun with or after the start of their CFS. This is about the same frequency of psychiatric disability seen in patients with other chronic illnesses. When we evaluated the degree of anger, depression, and anxiety in depressives and patients with CFS and MS, we found that the CFS and MS patients resembled one another in having fewer problems with each of these factors than was the case for the depressives.[31] Other studies have also found differences between depressives who do not have CFS and CFS patients who also are depressed. A major difference is the lack of guilt and self-blame in CFS patients.[32] Thus the risk of suicide, which is so great for the depressed patient, is very small for the CFS patient even when depressed.

We have recently compared depression scores in CFS patients with those reported by MS and depressed patients.[33] Again, the CFS patients resembled MS patients in having less self-reproach but more somatic symptoms than depressed patients. Results such as these seem to signify that CFS is not a variant of depression. The lack of efficacy of the antidepressant Prozac in a major clinical trial supports this interpretation.[34] This conclusion in no way negates the fact that CFS symptoms are worse when depression is also present.

The current activities at our center no longer exclude CFS patients because of their having had a psychiatric diagnosis prior to their illness. We simply use our diagnostic testing to determine whether or not that problem existed, and we plan to compare the two groups of CFS patients. Our purpose is to determine whether the illness is the same for the two groups or whether there are differences in the characteristics of the illness, its consequences, or its causes. We have learned that the vast majority of CFS patients with prior psychiatric problems have been sick for many years. This is quite different from patients who have had no prior emotional problems and suddenly developed CFS; many of these patients have been sick for only a few years. The members of this "CFS-prior psych" group may constitute a large number of patients who are chronically and severely ill; they may represent a great proportion of disabled people with chronic fatigue. In this regard, prior psychiatric problems seem to serve as another "illness amplifier."

What can we conclude from all this information pertaining to the notion that CFS is simply a form of depression? The most certain conclusion is that this idea does not hold for some CFS patients—namely, the group who have never had any evidence of depression. Without a definitive laboratory test for CFS, we simply cannot disentangle the relationship between depression, disease, and the demoralization that may accompany being chronically ill for those patients who have depression, either as part of their CFS or preceding it.

Analysis of Possible Causes

Without any definitive biomedical marker, our diagnostic capabilities remain at the clinical syndromal level. Discussions of "cause" tend to be based on opinion or point of view. We have dealt with the issue of depression; the remaining possibilities break down into three major groups: those who believe that CFS is a functional illness, those who believe that it is a medical illness, and those who believe that it is a combination of both.

Somatization Disorder

Let us begin with the idea that CFS is a functional illness, and turn to consideration of its being a manifestation of somatization disorder (SD).[35] Like other illnesses for which no diagnostic test exists, SD is diagnosed by case criteria that have been reached by consensus. The most rigorous case definition for a woman requires that she have a history of sickliness beginning before the age of thirty and at least thirteen physical complaints that are not believed to have a medical cause. A much more relaxed definition, used for studies of how frequently SD occurs in various communities, demands only six complaints that are not thought to have a medical cause. The sorts of complaints that a doctor might classify as nonmedical include abdominal pain, excessive gas, shortness of breath, dizziness, irregular or painful menstruation, and blurred vision. The physician relies on judgment to make this decision, and this clinical judgment may be right or wrong. Moreover, many of the symptoms in the somatization symptom list include those experienced by the CFS patient. Obviously, it is *critical* whether the examiner counts CFS symptoms as having a medical cause or not. Depending on which criterion we used and whether CFS symptoms were counted as medical or not, we were able to make the diagnosis of SD in either 2 percent or 98 percent of our carefully defined CFS patients![36] Thus, somatization disorder is simply too vague a construct to help in understanding chronic fatigue syndrome.

A number of researchers in Leeds, England, have looked at the SD question from a different viewpoint.[37] They reasoned that if CFS were a form of SD, one would expect to find substantially more abnormal illness behavior than in chronic illnesses in which the organic pathology is not in doubt. They compared illness behavior in patients with CFS and MS. Essentially the behavior in both groups was similar— highly abnormal when compared to healthy people—but showing no difference between CFS and MS. Thus this study does not confirm the SD hypothesis. Saying this does not eliminate the possibility that these symptoms are a somatic manifestation of emotional distress. Probably a subgroup of patients do have severe and chronic fatigue on this basis. The critical research question is how to support or prove this idea.

Hypochondriasis

Hypochondriasis is the cousin of somatization disorder. The hypochondriac worries about the possibility of becoming ill and is preoccupied with bodily functions. One point of view is that CFS is simply a form of hypochondriasis in which the individual worries about being ill without the existence of actual illness. A recent paper on hypochondriasis in CFS shows how flawed studies can lead to strong but probably untenable conclusions.[38] The researchers determined symptom count in a group of CFS patients and also asked them to complete questionnaires on hypochondriasis and on quality of life. Since the hypochondriasis questionnaire asked about physical illness and symptoms, it is not surprising that a firm relationship between physical symptom score and degree of hypochondriasis emerged. To my mind, this study does not advance our knowledge at all. Symptomatic patients are going to answer affirmatively to questions such as "Do you worry about your health more than other people?" and "Do you get the feeling that people are not taking your illness seriously enough?" Answering affirmatively does not mean the patient is a hypochondriac.

My interpretation is further supported by the Leeds study mentioned earlier. Both the MS and the CFS groups had high scores on a test of general hypochondriasis. Thus it seems inappropriate to use patients with unexplained illness for studies on hypochondriasis. Doing so makes the same degree of sense as evaluating such patients for somatization; the resulting circular argument does not move the field ahead. In order for us to know the true role of hypochondriasis in CFS, some researcher would have to do the hard experiment: administer the hypochondriasis questionnaire to a group of people who are at risk of getting CFS, but who do not have it at the time they complete the questionnaire. After some of these people did develop CFS, the researcher could determine if they had a hypochondriacal tendency *prior* to falling ill.

Meanwhile, the consequences of concluding that the relation between hypochondriasis and CFS symptom count is significant can lead to conclusions that are probably more wrong than right. For instance, the authors of the hypochondriasis study use the results to support their belief that the existence of CFS indicates endogenous depression and that aggressive treatment of this underlying psychiatric disorder will reduce the hypochondriasis and thence the symptoms. That is a large logical leap, which raises a lot of questions. What about the CFS patient with no apparent depression? Should she be treated as if she has hidden depression too? And if depression is such an important cause of CFS, why was a recent clinical trial using the well-known antidepressant Prozac not successful in alleviating any of the symptoms of the illness?[39] This example of circular thinking will remain with us until objective measures are developed to diagnose CFS.

Neurasthenia

What about the concept that CFS is a modern version of neurasthenia?[40] I find the evidence for this idea almost overwhelming. But saying that CFS is neurasthenia does not mean that CFS is a functional illness in the sense that people visualize when they discuss neurasthenia. Here again, the point is that the illness is "imagined" or "psychogenic." Even so, it is possible that careful testing will uncover some biomedical marker that can be used in the diagnosis and treatment of this disorder. Calling CFS a modern version of neurasthenia does not move our understanding further ahead.

Hyperventilation

Our group did find some evidence for hyperventilation in a preliminary study where patients had to breathe through a scuba diver–type mouthpiece while wearing nose clips.[41] However, when we repeated the study without mouthpiece and nose clips, we did not see signs of hyperventilation. Perhaps CFS patients are sensitive to the stress inherent in using mouthpiece and nose clips. If that turns out to be the case in later experiments, it may explain why CFS patients complain of being so stress sensitive. It will be important to determine this, because hyperventilation is treatable by breathing exercises or biofeedback.

Portrait of a Patient

Let me use the story of a "pretend" patient to move us toward other lines of thought on the cause of CFS. I should emphasize that this pretend patient resembles over 70 percent of the patients who have participated in the research activities of our New Jersey CFS Center. She is a Caucasian woman in her mid-thirties, previously in good health medically and psychologically. Although she may or may not have exercised regularly, she was a busy and active person—managing a family and a job at the same time. The woman is neither a "type" nor does she perform a "standard" kind of work. By this I mean that she can come from any social or economic stratum of our country and can work in any occupation, ranging from farming to clerical to professional to managerial.

When this patient comes to see me, she reports that her life was suddenly put on hold when she came down with a flu-like illness in which she had a fever, swollen and painful lymph glands in the neck, and a sore throat. Associated with this flu was sudden onset of fatigue and the other flu-like symptoms that constitute CFS. Unfortunately, her illness was not the flu, in that it did not go away. It remained for months or even years. Some days are relatively better than others. But in general, her activity is greatly limited. If she is still able to work, she does so by using all her sick time, by having an understanding boss, and by giving up any other life but work. If she is sicker and unable to work, she will be fighting to gain disability benefits while having to spend the bulk of her day at home resting or even sleeping.

Possible Infectious Agents

This story of sudden onset of illness in a previously healthy person and the flu-like symptoms of fever, sore throat, and painful lymph glands all suggest infection as a cause of CFS. Unfortunately, the hunt for a specific infectious agent has not yet been productive.

The history of the quest goes as follows. A group of scientists finds evidence via some sort of blood test that CFS patients, when compared to healthy people, have experienced an increased rate of a specific viral infection. The report of this finding is picked up by the media, which use headlines such as "Cause of CFS Found." The excitement generated tends to get in the way of the scientific process, because the path to knowledge begins to resemble a horse race, with different groups betting on different viruses that might cause the illness. Eventually, the talking dies down and the sleeves get rolled up. The large difference originally found between patients and controls inevitably tends to get smaller and smaller as results accumulate from more patients with CFS and other causes of fatiguing illness and from healthy controls. Things then stay quiet until a new positive result is found.

None of this is based on dishonesty; it is part of the scientific process. The chances for finding a difference in any measure between groups tends to be higher when the number of comparison groups and the size of the groups are small. Moreover, the scientific method demands that any finding be found repeatedly—not just by the group that made the original finding but by any group. In order to meet all these requirements, the finding must be relatively strong.

Viral Possibilities

Two viral families still have their adherents, and a third has just come to the attention of the medical community.

The Herpesviruses

The first is the class of viruses known to produce an acute infection and then go into hiding until something reactivates them and produces new symptoms. This is the herpesvirus family. I have already talked about the Epstein-Barr virus. Although some researchers still report results suggesting that EBV can reactivate in CFS, we have not found this in our own patients. Moreover, C. M. A. Swanink and her colleagues in the Netherlands actually calculated the load of virus in the blood of CFS patients and found it no different from that in healthy people.[42] This means that having mono (caused by the EBV) does not necessarily predispose to CFS. However, when one group of researchers looked only at a group of patients with mono, they did find that about 5 percent had fatigue that lasted more than six months;[43] half of these chronically fatigued patients had no psychiatric problems at all and fulfilled the more demanding 1988 case definition of CFS. Compared to the 0.1 percent prevalence of CFS in the community using that case definition, the rate of mono patients' developing CFS is high indeed!

A second herpesvirus, called human herpesvirus (HHV)-6, is an EBV look-alike that also causes infectious mononucleosis. Although the story on this virus is just developing, a number of studies suggest that it is active in the bodies of CFS patients at a higher rate than seen in healthy people.[44] The HHV-6 story has recently expanded to yet another newly discovered herpesvirus, human herpesvirus 7 (HHV-7); a recent report suggests that HHV-7, unlike HHV-6, occurs at high rates in both CFS patients and in healthy controls.[45] However, later in this chapter I will tell you about some encouraging results which suggest that a subgroup of CFS patients are positive for this virus more often than healthy controls.

Some preliminary evidence suggests that yet another herpesvirus might be involved in chronic fatigue syndrome. John Martin, a California pathologist, reported that he had isolated a virus resembling those of the herpesvirus family from a patient with CFS.[46] Whether or not that virus plays a role in the genesis of CFS demands the usual proof—a careful case control study in which specimens are assayed without any information about whether they came from patients or from controls.

The Enteroviruses

Because several outbreaks of CFS were reported to follow polio epidemics,[47] one idea was that the illness was a form of atypical polio. Thus attention was drawn to the family of viruses that causes polio— the enteroviruses. Although any possible tie between CFS and polio has been totally negated by continued cases of CFS in the absence of polio, a connection between one enterovirus, Coxsackie B, and CFS has been made. The tie was originally based on blood tests indicating evidence of prior infection, evidence that disappeared with larger numbers of patients and control subjects.[48] Still, one laboratory has reported finding the virus in muscle biopsies of CFS patients and not in muscle of healthy controls. Unfortunately, both a follow-up study by members of the original team and a separate study done by a different research team did not achieve the same result.[49] Probably, therefore, the enterovirus does not play an important role in generating the symptoms of CFS.

The Borna Disease Virus

In late 1996 attention turned to a new infectious agent, the Borna disease virus (BDV), previously thought to infect only animals. Workers in Osaka, Japan, found that psychiatric patients (most often suffering from depression) had antibodies indicating that they been infected by the virus seven times more often than healthy controls. Because psychiatric problems are common in CFS in Japan, the researchers then evaluated a CFS patient group. Of twenty-five CFS patients studied, 25 percent had evidence of prior infection in the form of antibodies in the blood, and an additional 9 percent actually had the virus detected in their white blood cells.[50] Unfortunately, these workers did not test for BDV in healthy controls. However, a prior study reported positivity in nearly 5 percent of healthy blood donors, a sevenfold difference from the CFS group. The difference in rates of positivity for patients and blood donors is impressive, but one would prefer to see control samples analyzed at the same time as patient samples.

My colleague James Dobbins also checked for BDV in twenty-five CFS patients and forty-six healthy controls, who were matched with the patients for age and sex. He found two positives in the patients and no positives in the controls. One notable difference between the two studies was that the majority of patients in the Japanese study were male, a very marked difference from the usual strong female prevalence reported in Euro-American CFS patients. My interpretation of these studies is that the BDV is a rare cause of CFS in Euro-American patients but may be more common in Japan and thus responsible for the gender differences noted in CFS patients there.

There is another possible explanation. The virus has been found in patients with major depression, and some CFS patients are depressed. Since neither the CDC nor the Osaka group divided their patients into those with and without psychiatric disorder, we cannot be sure that the virus was not tracking depression—rather than CFS. Obviously, those sorts of studies are in order.

The viral hypothesis lives, but since no specific virus has been found in nearly ten years of research, belief in it is waning. Perhaps the best evidence to support it is indirect. Robert Suhadolnik, a Philadelphia biochemist, has demonstrated that one of the body's antiviral defense mechanisms is turned on in CFS.[51] The inference is that a virus, or several viruses, have activated this mechanism. Should other groups confirm this finding, the marker of this antiviral process could become an important tag of viral activity in CFS. If so, Suhadolnik's work will support a role for viruses in the illness, but we still will not know specifically which ones.

Postinfectious Fatigue Syndrome
Because CFS seemed to follow an acute infectious process, patients who suddenly developed chronic fatigue and chronically present flu-

like symptoms were initially labeled as having postinfectious fatigue syndrome. A clear link between infection and CFS has not yet been made, so today all patients, regardless of how their illness begins, are given the diagnosis of CFS. However, since the workshop in the 1980s established the case definition for diagnosis and chose the name CFS, we have learned that three infectious illnesses can produce CFS: infectious mononucleosis, Lyme disease, and viral infection so severe as to require hospitalization.

The mononucleosis story is the best known and most fully described of the three. About 5 percent of mono patients never get better, develop excessive daytime sleepiness, and have all the complaints of a patient with CFS.[52] These patients do in fact have chronic mononucleosis, one of the earlier names for CFS. Although no one has ever applied the case definition to patients following infection with borrelia, the bacteria that cause Lyme disease, it seems clear that some patients, despite adequate treatment for their Lyme, continue to have symptoms of fatigue and widespread pain, and that these symptoms are consistent with the diagnosis of CFS. In one study, 31 percent of 114 borrelia-infected patients reported fatigue and joint pain without evidence of joint swelling many months after their initial diagnosis and treatment.[53] Moreover, the researchers reported that these patients often had many of the other symptoms consistent with the diagnosis of CFS.

The story of severe viral infection producing CFS is an interesting one. Studies by Simon Wessely and his colleagues in London specifically focused on viral meningitis because it is commonly caused by enteroviruses, and as I have indicated, the enteroviruses are one family of viruses thought to play a role in CFS. To increase their chance of finding a relationship between viral meningitis and CFS, the Wessely team decided to study only those patients who were sick enough to require hospitalization.[54] Comparison control patients were those with virus infection requiring hospitalization; cases of mono, hepatitis, and gastrointestinal enteroviral infection were specifically excluded because of the possibility that the viruses producing these illnesses could also produce CFS.

Six to twenty-four months after hospitalization, patients were surveyed via a questionnaire mailed to them. The researchers found no difference between the two groups in the rate of CFS but did find a very high rate of CFS in both—nearly 7 percent of the total. Thus, viral meningitis was not necessary for patients to develop CFS. The authors concluded that moderate to severe viral infections of any sort may play a part in the development of some cases of chronic fatiguing illness.

The fact that three infectious diseases can produce CFS supports the idea that chronic fatigue syndrome may be triggered by some other specific infectious agent. This information will certainly stimulate researchers to continue their search for such an agent. But the fact that no "specific" infectious cause has yet been found makes one pessimistic about its existence.

The Immunological Hypothesis

One very attractive alternative is that viral infection per se is not responsible for the clinical picture of CFS but instead that some such infection triggers a defective and extremely long-lived immune response. The past twenty years have produced an explosion of knowledge about the workings of the immune system. One important realization has been that it is not infection by bacteria or viruses that makes us sick, but rather the body's immunological response to the presence of the foreign material in the pathogen. The purpose of the immune system is to wipe out infection by foreign invaders such as bacteria or viruses. It does this by starting a chain reaction of responses in the white blood cells.

We all know that blood comprises both white and red cells, and because there are millions more red cells than white cells, the color of the blood is red. Red cells carry oxygen throughout the body, and white cells defend the body from foreign invaders. These white cells basically remain in a resting or waiting stage until they detect the presence of material that is immunologically different from the body's cells. Sensing these antigens produces a change in the form and function of the white blood cells. As activated white cells, they release tiny amounts of different substances called cytokines, which are links in the chain reaction whose purpose is to wipe out the foreign invaders. However, these cytokines make one sick; they are responsible for the fever and flu-like symptoms that accompany viral infection. Thus it is reasonable to conceptualize CFS as a problem of immunological control.

Unfortunately, the supporting evidence is not straightforward.[55] Some researchers have found small but seemingly real differences in some measures of cytokine activity; others, including our center, have been unable to replicate these results. Despite choosing criteria to select a rather homogeneous group of patients with CFS, we could find no specific abnormality in cytokines in our CFS patient population.

Coincident with the secretion of these cytokines is a change in the white blood cells themselves as they become immunologically activated. Again, some researchers have found differences in the numbers of activated white blood cells between CFS patients and healthy controls; but efforts of other laboratories, including our own, to replicate these findings have not been successful. More consistent results follow tests of the functioning white cells. In general, when the white cells of CFS patients are stimulated, they do not function as well as the white cells of healthy controls.

Why these results are so inconsistent remains ambiguous. Certainly one problem is the definition of CFS. But even with our center's definition, chosen to select the most consistent population of patients (frequently disabled and often homebound), we have been unable to replicate any of these immunological results despite great care with our immunological methods. Nevertheless, we have come up with an approach that looks promising.

The Splitter's Approach to CFS

Our center has adopted a further extension of the syndromic approach. We reasoned that the discrepancies across studies might reflect the fact that CFS was the clinical manifestation of an illness with more than one cause. Since we were most interested in finding a group of patients with a medical cause of CFS, one of our strategies was to separate our patients into two groups; the technical term is "stratify." One group comprised patients without evidence of psychiatric illness at any time in their lives. The second group was composed of CFS patients who had a psychiatric illness that had begun at or after the onset of their CFS. We hypothesized that we would find differences between these groups. Specifically, we thought we might find immunological or viral abnormalities in the first group but not in the second.

The problem with the "splitter's" approach is that with each split, the number of patients available for analysis is halved, so the researcher must recruit twice as many subjects in order to have a reasonable number in each group. Although we are currently dealing with that problem, we have already gotten some tantalizing results that support our thinking. Because of the CFS patient's frequent complaint of difficulties with concentration and memory, we have done large-scale neuropsychological testing to compare cognitive function in CFS patients to that in healthy controls. In our overall group of CFS patients, we did find problems in cognitive function, but they were minor in comparison to the severity of the patients' complaints.[56] One important finding was that the patients with cognitive impairment were more disabled, as evidenced by more inactivity in the form of more time in bed, than those with normal cognitive function.

Further insight into what was happening required that we divide the patients into our two groups.

The CFS group with no psychiatric diagnosis had significantly worse cognitive dysfunction, a finding that clearly separated CFS from depression.[57] Depression is known to produce cognitive problems, but the individuals in this particular CFS group had no evidence of depression. Why, then, did they have cognitive impairment? My diagnostic impression was that this group of patients had a brain problem. To a neurologist such as me, cognitive dysfunction occurring in an otherwise healthy person without explanation indicates that something is wrong with the brain; the term for this is "encephalopathy."

In our study, those who appeared to have an encephalopathy were the patients who were normal one day, suddenly fell sick with CFS the next day, then remained ill without any concurrent psychiatric problems. That pattern supported our thinking that the cause was some viral or immunological problem. Although we had found no differences in viral or immunological data over our entire CFS group, we do have preliminary evidence for one cytokine being at lower levels in this group than in healthy sedentary women. Similarly, we find that the CFS group with no psychiatric diagnosis is more often positive for both HHV-6 *and* HHV-7 infection than either the patient group who also had a psychiatric diagnosis or the healthy sedentary group. Certainly we need to continue collecting data to increase our patient numbers in each group, but it is fascinating that our information thus far supports our use of the syndromic approach and our tactic of being splitters.

Brain Dysfunction
Several other pieces of information point toward the idea that some patients with CFS may have a neurological illness affecting their brain. Unfortunately, little of that work has used the splitter's approach, so questions remain.

In the first study, my colleagues and I evaluated brain magnetic resonance images on fifty-two CFS patients and fifty-two people who were imaged for headache or minor head injury. In contrast to X-rays, which allow the doctor to see the skull but not the brain within, magnetic resonance imaging (MRI) allows one to see also the structures of the brain—noninvasively. This huge medical advance was based on the fact that different anatomic structures in the brain are composed of varying amounts of water, and the magnet can be tuned to "see" water.

In contrast to the one patient in the comparison group who had an abnormality, we found fourteen CFS patients to have abnormalities.[58] These were of two types. The first, seen in nine patients, consisted of small, circular bright-appearing areas not normally seen in MR images except those of elderly people and individuals with vascular disease. Several years after the initial neurological examination, I recontacted these patients and learned that the doctors of three of them believed their fatiguing illness might have a medical cause such as multiple sclerosis. For the remaining five patients, CFS remained the diagnosis.

The second type of abnormality, seen in five patients, consisted of enlarged fluid-containing spaces in the brain. For the fluid space to enlarge, there must be a loss of brain tissue, atrophy. Since other researchers have reported the first abnormality but not the second, we are currently repeating this work by imaging our carefully evaluated CFS patients from the Center.

One condition that could mimic our MRI findings is mild traumatic brain injury (MTBI). Trauma to the brain can kill brain cells; if enough die, one can see atrophy with fluid spaces enlarged to compensate for the loss of brain substance. We had not screened for MTBI in the original study, but we routinely do so in our current Center research protocols. If our project finds evidence of enlarged fluid spaces in CFS patients who have no other explanation for loss of brain tissue, the results will support the idea that some CFS patients have a neurological illness.

Although we are not at the point of confirming this theory, preliminary results on the first type of brain MR abnormality again support the splitter's approach. Our study is not complete, but we are finding no difference in the rate of abnormalities between healthy controls and patients who developed a psychiatric illness after their CFS began. Significantly, the CFS group devoid of major psychiatric problems had many more lesions than the other two groups. (Let me remind you that this is the group with the greatest problem on tests of attention and memory, as well as the group with the highest rate of positivity to the HHV-6 and HHV-7 viruses.) The fact that we are finding different abnormalities in the same CFS patient subgroup points to that group as being the one with brain dysfunction—caused perhaps by an as-yet-undiscovered virus or an immunologically active agent.

Abnormal Hypothalamo-Pituitary-Adrenal Function
Other information does exist to support the idea that there is a brain abnormality in CFS. That conclusion is based on studies of the hypothalamopituitary axis. The hypothalamus in the brain has many diverse functions. Among these is control of a small pea-sized organ called the pituitary gland. Neural traffic from higher centers activates groups of nerve cells or neurons in the hypothalamus. These cells release hormones into the blood vessels that bathe the pituitary gland, and these hormones activate other hormonal systems in that gland.

The pituitary gland is known as the master gland in the body because its hormonal secretions control other hormonal glands. Hormones released by the pituitary enter the bloodstream to influence the thyroid gland, the adrenal gland, and the reproductive organs (the testicles and the ovaries).

The first study looked at the brain's control of adrenal function and found it somewhat impaired.[59] The results were the opposite from those seen in depression. Instead of the activation of the hypothalamo-pituitary-adrenal axis that occurs in depressed people, CFS patients showed reduced activity of this axis. This finding immediately produced interest, because reduced adrenal function—a condition known as Addison's disease—is characterized by severe fatigue. Many doctors have tried treating CFS patients with steroids, stronger versions of the natural adrenal hormones, without much success.

So although it appears that CFS is not a result of reduced cortisol secretion by the adrenal gland, the results still point to some problem in control by the hypothalamus of pituitary-adrenal hormone secretion. Supporting this notion is a report from Australia, in which a biomedical marker was found in the urine of CFS patients; this marker resembled a brain-active drug known to alter the hypothalamo-pituitary-adrenal axis.[60] However, an alternative explanation has recently been advanced for the "abnormality."[61] A group of endocrinologists, experts on hormones and organs that secrete hormones, studied pituitary-adrenal hormone levels in a group of nurses who had worked the night shift for five days. The doctors, finding the same picture of impaired adrenal function in the nurses as had been reported in the CFS patients, explained the adrenal problem in the CFS patients as simply caused by disrupted sleep and social routine.

Disrupted Sleep and Stress
The idea that disrupted sleep may have endocrinological consequences is reinforced by a study done on patients with fibromyalgia, which, when present with fatigue, reflects severe chronic fatigue syndrome. In normal people, sleep causes the pituitary gland to secrete growth hormone, which plays an important role in muscle growth and repair from injury. Patients with FM had lower levels of a growth-hormone—related substance called somatomedin.[62] Whether this endocrine abnormality merely reflects disrupted sleep or acts somehow

to produce muscle tenderness is not known, but the hormone study on the nurses points toward the first explanation. The Boston CFS Center has found the same "abnormality" in a group of CFS patients. One wonders whether sleep-disrupted healthy people would have the urinary abnormality noted from Australia.

Although this work does not clearly implicate the hypothalamus in producing CFS, other evidence exists for dysfunction in this part of the brain in CFS. One way of increasing neural traffic to the hypothalamus is to induce stress, routinely done in the laboratory by injecting insulin intravenously. Insulin causes muscle cell membranes to open to allow entry of glucose, the most common blood sugar. Glucose levels in the blood then fall, so the brain, which has a continual need for glucose, detects the lowered levels and produces the state of stress. People with low blood sugar feel anxious, tremulous, and sweaty. An additional response is activation of the pituitary gland.

When CFS patients, stratified to exclude those with any history of psychiatric problems, and healthy controls underwent this insulin-induced stress, the pituitary response in the patient group was impaired.[63] Our group has just completed its own stress study. Instead of using insulin, we produced stress by asking patients and controls to walk quickly on an ever-increasing incline until they could walk no further. In response to that stimulus, pituitary as well as some aspects of adrenal function of CFS patients was impaired compared to controls.

Exposure to Pesticides
A final idea on the possibility that CFS produces brain dysfunction comes from preliminary studies on the role of pesticides.[64] Since toxin exposure is known to produce many symptoms resembling CFS, a patient reporting an unambiguous association between exposure to pesticides and the development of chronic fatigue would not be diagnosed as having CFS; the diagnosis would be low-dose toxin exposure.

However, an Australian group hypothesized that perhaps some people were exposed to toxic amounts of insecticide unknowingly, and that it was this exposure which produced their CFS. They supported this hypothesis by finding evidence in the blood suggestive of toxic exposure in the patient group but not in healthy controls. An important next step will be to see if other groups can replicate this potentially important finding.

The weight of all these studies certainly points to a brain problem in at least some CFS sufferers. If other evidence continues to support this interpretation, it will indeed mean that some CFS patients have an encephalopathy. The term "myalgic encephalopathy" may thus be an appropriate one—at least for some patients with CFS.

Muscle Abnormalities

In contrast to the idea that CFS might originate from a problem in the brain is the idea that it might originate from a problem in the muscles. Obviously, if the muscles do not work correctly, they will easily become fatigued. And this is what happens in myasthenia. Unfortunately, the evidence for true muscle dysfunction is unclear. Tests of muscle strength, the time to fatigue, and the response of muscle to electrical stimulation have all shown no differences between CFS patients and healthy controls.

The best evidence for CFS patients having a problem in their muscles is based on muscle biopsy.[65] Researchers in Liverpool, England, have reviewed the work of other groups and have done their own evaluation of biopsies of twenty-two healthy people and seventy-four CFS patients, fifty-six of whom had muscle pain. Abnormalities were found in 32 percent of healthy people and in 81 percent of CFS patients, and as often in CFS patients in whom muscle pain was not a prominent complaint as in patients with that complaint. The abnormalities seen in both healthy people and CFS patients were of varied types, suggesting that the findings were not specific to CFS. Still, the strikingly large number of abnormalities in the CFS group is impressive.

Our group has performed an experiment to look at muscle function. Like the brain imaging study discussed earlier, it uses the technology of magnetic resonance. But instead of targeting the brain's water to provide images of the brain, the technique targets the phosphate ion—a different constituent of every living cell. The phosphate ion is key to normal cellular function. When we do things, muscle cells use glucose as an energy source to contract and allow us to do what we wish. Via the actions of insulin, glucose enters the muscle cell and is used by it to energize phosphate ions. When a phosphate ion is charged with energy, it attaches to another substance called creatine to make the high-energy substance phosphocreatine. When we call our muscles into action, the phosphocreatine gives up its energy to make the muscle fiber contract; phosphate and creatine are left behind. Magnetic resonance spectroscopy (MRS) can tell us how much phosphocreatine and how much phosphate is present in any muscle, without the need for a muscle biopsy. This information tells us about the bioenergetics of muscle—noninvasively.

My colleague Kevin McCully is expert in the technique of MRS. To learn about muscle bioenergetics in CFS as compared to sedentary healthy controls, we performed MRS on the calf muscle on a baseline day, and again no more than two days after a stress test in which subjects were asked to walk quickly on a progressively greater incline until they could not walk any more. The results were surprising.[66] Basically, the bioenergetics of the patients was the same both times as that of the sedentary controls. Since muscle injury alters the bioenergetic pattern of MRS, the results indicated that microtrauma to muscle was not responsible for the CFS patients' complaint of marked post-exertional fatigue.

In addition to evaluating bioenergetics in the resting state, McCully studied bioenergetics during work—while subjects pressed their foot up and down on a weighted pedal. Since he could see the muscles use phosphocreatine, McCully could tell all patients to stop working at the same time, when their calf muscle had used up a certain proportion of available high-energy phosphate. Again, there was no difference in the amount of time to reach the stopping point. But when McCully calculated the time it took for the muscle to restore its levels of high-energy phosphocreatine, he did find a difference. The patients achieved this much more slowly than did the sedentary controls. When a muscle physiologist finds this result, he is apt to diagnose a problem with the muscle cell itself.

Problems of Integrating the Results

It is time to back up and try to put all this information together. How can we explain these variable results? True, the evidence is persuasive that CFS may involve the brain of some patients, but what about our study of muscle bioenergetics? How about the viral and immunological work? Why do some laboratories find biomedical markers of CFS while others cannot?

One answer has to do with what statisticians call sampling. When researchers study twenty patients and twenty controls, they hope that each group is representative of the much larger group of all CFS patients and all healthy controls. Occasionally this is not the case. That was my explanation for our failure to replicate our finding that CFS patients had been exposed to much more stress prior to their illness than a comparison group of healthy controls. A second answer has to do with stratification, with trying to sort the pool of all CFS patients into intelligently conceived subgroups.

Comparison Groups

Yet another possible reason for the difficulty in finding a consistent biomedical marker or abnormal test for identification of CFS is that discrepancies may exist because of the comparison groups chosen. The study of hypothalamo-pituitary-adrenal function of the nurses working night shifts makes this point clearly.[67] A major complaint of the CFS patient is unrefreshing sleep. When the sleep of the nurses was disrupted by their having to work night shifts, they showed the same hormonal changes as in CFS. The scientists concluded that the "hormonal dysfunction" was due not to disease but to disrupted sleep. Their conclusion emphasizes the possibility of problems in choosing comparison groups in order to identify biomedical markers. In this specific study, healthy people were in all likelihood not the right comparison group. What would have been the right group?

Inactivity

Chronic fatigue syndrome carries with it one effect that could greatly complicate our understanding of its causes; that effect is inactivity. These patients rest a great deal during their day. In fact, the original case definition of CFS required patients to reduce their activity by at least 50 percent relative to their activity levels prior to onset. And inactivity carries its own baggage. First, it makes people less fit, so almost any effort makes them short of breath and fatigued. Next, it makes them dizzy when they stand up. This kind of posture-related dizziness is called orthostatic instability. In 1995 a group at Johns Hopkins University reported that CFS patients frequently have orthostatic instability.[68] They put CFS patients on a tilt table and left them tilted three-quarters of the way up for many minutes. A large number complained of feeling faint. In our experience, healthy people respond in this way too, and probably would do so more often if asked to go to bed for several days beforehand. Finally, inactivity alters immune function.

The question, then, is, Are the exertional fatigue, orthostatic instability, and immunological abnormalities of CFS markers of the illness, or are they present because CFS has made the patient inactive, requiring a lot of bedrest?

How to answer this question? We could ask a lot of healthy people to become inactive, but for how long and how inactive? The parameters are just too vague. How about the opposite tactic? We could see if CFS patients can be made more fit by gentle aerobic training. As I will detail in a later chapter, we have tried this fitness training as part of our rehabilitation approach and some patients swear by it. They claim it reduces their fatigue and their pain. But we have only their opinion that training reduces their symptoms. We are performing a more definitive study that will determine whether CFS patients can follow a training program, whether training relieves CFS symptoms, and whether lack of fitness is responsible for some of the "abnormalities" that have been found. To obtain this last result, we will have to see the so-called abnormalities disappear as the CFS patient's fitness improves. If we do find this result, it will allow us to understand the discrepancies in results from one CFS center to the next. The experts in CFS can then start anew to try to understand the cause of this disabling illness.

We have reason to be optimistic about the outcome of our trial, based on information coming from London researchers since 1995. One outcome study noted less functional impairment in patients who attempted to maintain some level of activity.[69] Peter White, who has completed a study much like the one we are currently doing, has found that aerobic conditioning produces lasting improvement compared to a treatment of stretching exercises accompanied by muscle relaxation. Even eighteen months after the conditioning program, thirty-five of forty-seven patients continued to rate themselves improved, and many had returned to the activity levels they had exhibited prior to their illness. The critical question we hope to answer is what happens to the biomedical markers of CFS after such a conditioning trial.

Current Formulations and Long-Term Outlook

If indeed viral and immunological markers, cognitive dysfunction, and abnormal muscle bioenergetics return to normal after such a trial, what can we invoke as the cause of chronic fatigue syndrome? Simon Wessely, a London psychiatrist and epidemiologist, believes that a vicious cycle of progressive loss of fitness and fear of exertion may be the explanation.[70] The formulation is as follows. An individual develops a flu-like illness where physical exertion produces a worsening of all symptoms. The patient decides that the only recourse is to rest more and exert less. This pattern leads to a progressive loss of fitness such that even minor effort produces much worse fatigue as well as the other CFS symptoms. The reaction reinforces the patient's unwillingness to exert herself and in fact may make her afraid to do so. Fitness tumbles, muscles atrophy, and fear of trying increases. The reasonableness of this formulation is evidenced by the fact that treatments to break up this vicious cycle make the CFS patient better.

Before concluding this chapter, let me give another, rather different idea of the identity of CFS. I have laid out the argument that it is an abnormal condition, not experienced by normal people: an individual either does or does not have the illness (cancer being an easily understood example). But an alternative point of view is that CFS is simply an extreme of normal human experience.

In fact, information exists to support this thesis. One group mailed questionnaires on the existence and magnitude of fatigue to more than thirty thousand people registered in medical practices in southern England.[71] Of the over fifteen thousand people who responded, nearly six thousand reported substantial fatigue, and half of the responders claimed to have had it for six months or longer. The researchers concluded by suggesting that CFS "may represent a morbid excess of fatigue rather than a discrete entity, just as high blood pressure and alcohol consumption are morbid ends of normal spectrums." A similar argument has recently been made for the pain of fibromyalgia.[72]

Although these arguments are certainly reasonable for substantial fatigue and pain, whether or not they pertain to the "fatigue plus" that constitutes CFS remains ambiguous. If further research efforts do not identify a reliable laboratory abnormality in CFS (when compared to appropriate groups), the notion that CFS is an extreme of the normal human experience with fatigue and pain will gain credence. However, the research will have to change focus to determine why some people are apparently at higher risk of developing this problem than others.

It is obvious that our knowledge of what causes CFS is hazy. Working to clarify difficult problems of this sort is the thrill of research. But our lack of knowledge about causes does not imply a lack of treatment. As you will see, the medical profession is often able to help patients despite its ignorance of what produces the symptoms or the illness.

5 ⟨ Understanding the Doctor

Before we move on to the treatments available for fatigue, it is critical that we deal with the problem faced by many patients with severe and chronic fatigue when they go to the doctor. I cannot count the times patients have told me that I am the twelfth or the fifteenth doctor they consulted, and of their frustration during those earlier contacts. Why is there so often a problem in communication between patients with severe fatigue and their doctors?

Often doctors and patients have different agendas, which are not communicated to the other party. I have written a book for aspiring doctors that warns them of this problem,[1] but one small book is no cure. Understanding the reasons for the communication gap is critical to ensure the fullest attention of your doctor and, as a consequence, the best care. Achieving this goal will require that you understand the doctor's agenda.

Among the troublesome factors for the doctor in communicating with patients are an understanding of what the job comprises and something I call medical materialism.

The Physician's Job

Doctors-in-training are rarely told in so many words what their function is. Because of this remarkable lapse in the teaching of medicine, doctors tend to make up their own explanations of their role. Basically, a doctor's job depends very strongly on whether the individual is a *physician* or a *surgeon*. My use of these words, which date from the 1700s, is very specific. A surgeon is someone who is extremely procedure driven, whereas a physician tends to be very patient driven. So a surgeon can naturally enough be a person with scalpel in hand whose job it is to remove an infected appendix or a cancer. But my definition would also give the surgeon label to groups of very different types of doctors. For instance, an emergency-room doctor is driven by procedures to move people out of the emergency room—either back home or into a hospital room. Reversing calamities is this doctor's middle name. So when patients come in bleeding from an open wound or blue in color because they have stopped breathing, this doctor does what has to be done to get things back to normal. He or she acts as a surgeon would. In other words, the job of the surgeon is to cure. The curing may be done in pretty much the same way it has been done for centuries—by cutting out—but many surgical techniques are new and sophisticated.

If the surgeon's job is to cure, what is the physician's job? It is to help. That is, the physician's job is to hold the patient's hand in one hand and the family's hand in the other, and to walk through time with patient and family during the course of the patient's illness.

What is missing from this description is the word "cure." Although the field of medicine has made huge amounts of progress in developing tests to aid in diagnosing specific diseases, relatively little progress has been made in advancing our understanding of what causes those diseases. And when we do know the cause, we do not know how to prevent the disease from occurring.

Therefore, the number of diseases a physician can cure is very small. The physician can cure vitamin deficiencies such as scurvy or beriberi. The physician can cure hormone deficiencies such as a low thyroid state. The physician can cure bacterial infections like a strep throat. The physician can cure fungal infections like ringworm or athlete's foot. We are beginning to see drugs that can cure the rare viral infection. And, astonishingly, the physician can cure an occasional cancer. In diseases such as heart failure or Alzheimer's disease or most cancers, the doctor is unable to *cure,* but instead can *help* the patient cope with the symptoms produced.

We return to the problem that arises between patients and doctors. Often the doctor has not realized that the job is not to cure but to help. The word "help" has no borders: anything that makes the patient feel better is allowed. The physician's first remedy is the pharmacopeia—the pharmacological option. Take the common cold as an example. Unable to cure it, the physician can nonetheless prescribe medicines that lessen the symptoms and allow the sufferer to feel better. The same principle holds for epilepsy, heart failure, and most other diseases—including cancer.

Physicians get a bit uncomfortable if the pharmacological option does not work and the patient still needs help. A new option that they are just learning to call on is rehabilitation medicine, a specialty devoted to helping patients cope with long-term disabilities. Originally, the area dealt predominantly with loss of limb by amputation, or organ of sensation as in loss of vision. But the field of rehabilitation medicine is now open to people disabled by any disease. The combination of creative thinking and the burgeoning of the computer era has brought help via ramps and rails for people with gait unsteadiness, to voice-operated programs for use in communicating on computer bulletin boards to people unable to move because of a broken neck. Today's physicians must be creative and generate options to help each patient on a case-by-case basis.

The Molding Process

Another type of communication problem between physician and patient is a peculiar type of molding that begins in medical school and moves into high gear during postgraduate training. This molding process has to do with the particular qualities and personality of the medical student, the pressures in the student's life, and his or her colleagues and peers. The medical student who is focused and mature can avoid being molded. Unfortunately, the youth and relative inexperience of most medical students make them highly susceptible to the peer pressure that changes a considerate young doctor-to-be into someone who can be described by the 3 Bs—brash, boorish, and bullying—in addition to being unkind and a poor listener.

Although medical schools are trying to change focus from the technical to the personal, the way they are organized and the extreme emphasis on technical skills and knowledge tend to mold medical students into people different from what they were upon entry. Medical schools, like other large organizations, tend to have departments with more and more specialized functions. The reason for this division is to organize and teach the vast body of medical knowledge students need in order to learn the facts of medicine. In the first two years of medical education, students are taught to think about the human body as parsed into a number of discrete chunks: first in terms of its normal structure and function, later in terms of the changed structure and function that are characteristic of disease. Because of the "fact load," time is not available to help the student synthesize the facts of medicine. Thus, the individual pieces become all important. Except for the rare young doctor who realizes that the whole is more important than its parts and who has both the time and the intelligence to put the pieces together to better understand the whole patient, most young doctors think it adequate to know only the facts of medicine. Thus the curriculum forces into the student a bias in favor of technology and against communication and empathy.

This process of focusing on individual facts picks up speed in the last two years of medical school, when the curriculum turns to teaching the student how to diagnose and deal with disease. The "focusing down" process goes hand-in-hand with the tendency to make specialists out of many medical students. Again, the fact load seems to be what produces this specialization, the divisions of cardiology, gastroenterology, dermatology, nephrology, and many others in a typical medical school department of medicine. Each of these divisions is further subdivided by the fact load and the techniques available to help produce the information needed to decide what the facts are— that is, to be able to diagnose the patient's problem. As an example, one new subspecialty is interventional cardiology; physicians choosing this area learn the techniques needed to thread tiny catheters into tiny vessels within the heart, to allow them to be seen or opened up if they are clogged by arteriosclerotic disease. Opting for such a strategy is self-protective for several reasons. It makes it possible for an individual doctor to know all there is to know about the field. And because of the doctor's ability to know all the facts in the field, it protects him or her—as much as is possible—from the threat of malpractice suits, which are a frequent worry for the practitioner.

Thus, this approach tends to be extremely fact oriented and not very patient oriented. Again, only the unusual medical student is able to find the time and mental energy to put these facts in perspective and to figure out how to apply them to a sick human being.

The final element that hastens this molding process is the medical student's financial worries. Medical students and law students share one characteristic: in contrast to graduate students in other disciplines, they must pay for their education. While debts of over $100,000 still tend to be somewhat uncommon, those of $50,000 are frequent. When your wardrobe is sneakers and jeans, a debt of $50,000 to $100,000 looms as enormous and is very frightening to face.

Confronted with this worry, students find out quickly that reimbursement is usually best for surgeons and for physicians who choose the more technical aspects of medicine. The student who originally wanted to be a family doctor has been subtly pushed to become an interventional cardiologist.

The advent of managed care is changing medicine in the United States and will have a strong impact on this molding process. Almost every medical professional understands that we are creating too many specialists and not enough generalists. In addition, the costs of medicine are very high; to make them more reasonable, the way doctors are paid will have to change. These messages have been filtering down to the students. For ten years, when I asked students what kind of medicine they hoped to practice, they answered with plans to become specialists and subspecialists. In the past few years, however, I have heard more and more say they want to become generalists. Why? Because with the development of health maintenance organizations (HMOs) and other new ways to deliver medical care, specialists today are finding it hard to locate jobs.

Anesthesiology, the specialty of putting people to sleep before surgery and making sure they wake up afterward, provides the best example. In the past, many medical students wanted to become anesthesiologists because the pay was stupendous. But HMOs need to cut costs. To do this, they hire one anesthesiologist to supervise the work of a group of nurse anesthetists, because nurses cost less to hire than physicians. Because of this rapid change, some anesthesiologists cannot find jobs, and anesthesiology training programs are suddenly shrinking. So market forces are pushing the medical student to enter the fields of family medicine or internal medicine, which will enable him or her to practice general medicine. Both fields demand postgraduate training years so that young doctors can learn what is needed to cope with patient complaints. Of the two fields, family medicine provides a broader perspective, which increases the chance that a doctor-in-training can put the facts together.

Medical Materialism

Simply becoming a generalist does not necessarily make a doctor better able to cope with unexplained illness like chronic fatigue syndrome or fibromyalgia or to listen when patients cite vague complaints such as fatigue or pain throughout the body. Even generalists often have poor communications skills. Once again, the problem of medical materialism arises from the medical school's focus on facts. By medical materialism I mean the doctor's reliance on abnormal laboratory tests or pathology. A surprising thing often occurs when doctors cannot hold an abnormal test result in their hands: they tend to think there is nothing wrong with the patient. Some doctors make the odd assumption that if they know all the facts about an illness, they know all there is to know about that illness. Obviously, this assumption is mistaken because at any particular point in time we only know what we know.

Schizophrenia, a disease synonymous with insanity, illustrates how the facts of medicine change. For several generations, this terrible illness was thought to be caused by psychological factors and treatable by psychotherapy. No brain abnormality could ever be found, either by lab test or on the autopsy table. Now medical research has shown that schizophrenia is a disease and not just a reaction to stress. The disease is inherited and produces abnormalities that can be seen in brain imaging tests and in biochemical analyses of brain tissue.

Unfortunately, if the teacher does not emphasize this fact to the medical student, medical materialism develops and the patient suffers. First the doctor assures himself or herself that nothing is wrong with the patient, then gets angry at the patient for taking up part of a busy day, and finally rejects the patient and the patient's complaints—sometimes quite impolitely. Thus medical materialism joins the other forces that mold the young doctor into someone who does not hear what the patient is saying.

Doctor-Patient Expectations

The final piece of the equation that leads to poor understanding between doctor and patient lies in the realm of expectations.[2] Doctors' ears tend to perk up when they hear what they expect, and droop when what they hear means nothing to them. Again, this reflects what the doctors have been taught. If a patient comes to the doctor complaining of coughing up blood, that complaint is so obviously abnormal that it galvanizes the physician's attention. If, on the other hand, the patient complains of incredible fatigue, that complaint is so common and applicable to so many situations that it often goes ignored. Something that is of major importance to the patient is not heard by the doctor. Instead, the doctor continues trying to get information that makes medical sense to him or her. And once again, if the doctor cannot make medical sense out of the history, he or she assumes that the problem is psychological, that there is nothing wrong with the patient, and that the patient should not be wasting the doctor's time. The patient is left to figure out what to do next.

From this discussion, it is evident that medical school prepares the young physician to deal with diagnosable problems. Because this group of illnesses is so large, there is little time to teach the physician how to deal with unexplained illnesses and complaints. So when the physician sees such a patient, it is a frustrating experience because he or she lacks "tools" to deal with the individual. When the patient with unexplained illness has a difficult and demanding personality and/or a coexisting psychiatric disorder, the problems in establishing a satisfactory relationship are multiplied. More than 10 percent of physician contacts are with such patients.[3] Recognizing the reasons why interactions between doctors and patients are not always smooth is the first step toward remedying this problem. But you as a patient with unexplained symptoms need to understand why friction may exist between you and your doctor: your expectations may be basically different.

If such a conflict exists in the first or second doctor-patient meeting, you may find that you have made no headway in understanding your symptoms. And not knowing what is wrong makes the whole illness worse. Nearly every patient who has had this happen has thanked me when I have made the diagnosis of chronic fatigue syndrome, even though that diagnosis points to a severe and disabling illness. If such a patient does not find a physician who will say "The buck stops here," that person will move to alternative types of medicine—from chiropractic to homeopathy. Understanding the doctor is the first step in dealing with the doctor.

6 ɕ Problems with Sleep

Everyone experiences fatigue. And for the most part, we survive it quite well. The body is, after all, built to deal with stresses and strains; if troubles arise that interfere with sleep for a few days, fatigue puts you to bed to allow you to recover. Sometimes, however, the causes of fatigue are not transient. Or sometimes your efforts to deal with fatigue make it worse. Or occasionally your fatigue has a medical cause. In each of these cases, the body cannot adjust itself to the problem. The fatigue becomes more severe and more frequent—so much so, in fact, that it tends to be present all the time.

In this chapter we will begin to develop ways of dealing with fatigue. Specifically, we will focus on insomnia or nonrefreshing sleep, then in later chapters deal with other causes of fatigue.

Poor Sleep Hygiene

One guarantee of fatigue is poor sleep hygiene, poor habits related to going to bed. One can awake from sleep feeling refreshed, or toss and turn and awake exhausted; and it is possible to go from one extreme to the other. Eating late, drinking too much alcohol or coffee, or becoming accustomed to sedatives can all disturb sleep for some people. When you eat a large meal later than you usually do, the digestive processes can interfere with your sleep, most commonly via heartburn. Fluid in the stomach is acidic in order to begin the digestive process. Normally the mixture of food and gastric juice stays in the stomach, where it is slowly passed along into the intestine for further digestion. A fold at the top of the stomach usually prevents gastric juice from backing up into the esophagus, the tube that connects the mouth and the stomach. If you lie down with a full stomach, though, it is not unusual for some of the stomach's contents to back up into the esophagus. Since the lining of the esophagus is not protected from acid as is the lining of the stomach, this regurgitation results in heartburn. The degree of gastric reflux or regurgitation varies. Some people get the symptoms of heartburn or pressure in the chest when they go to bed, even if they have eaten many hours earlier.

An obvious way around this problem is to eat earlier, so that your food is digested before you are ready for bed. If that does not help, you can try taking antacids, which are available over the counter. There are two kinds of antacids, the old-fashioned kind that neutralizes the acid (Mylanta or Maalox) or the newer variety that stops the stomach from making the acid (Tagamet-AC). If one type does not work, the other may. Another suggestion is that you raise the head of your bed up a few inches by putting books under two legs. (Raising your head with pillows bends you in the middle and can make the problem worse.) One or a combination of these solutions should prevent your heartburn and allow you to achieve restful sleep.

Alcohol, often a part of our normal diet, is a drug that often has unexpected consequences. You can be a steady moderate drinker for many years, having a martini before dinner every night. Your body's ability to deal with alcohol can change with age, though. Whereas previously the drink may have had little effect, it can become sedating or even disturb your sleep. Omitting the drink for one or two nights really does not test whether the alcohol is disturbing your sleep; you have to limit your alcohol intake to one glass of wine per day for at least two weeks to determine if your sleep is more restful.

The same is true for coffee, which contains a drug that is a major stimulant and stomach acid secretor. Everyone knows that caffeine wakes you up. Too much of it can make you jumpy and give you heartburn. My rule of thumb is no coffee after noon. That gives plenty of time for the caffeine to be eliminated from your system. But this might not be the case if you drink ten cups of coffee before noon; in that case you will also have to cut back on the *amount* you consume. Remember, too, that coffee is not the only source of caffeine. It is found in tea, cola drinks, and chocolate. Again, if you have trouble sleeping, you need to cut back on these substances.

The warning holds for prescribed sedative-type drugs, too. Fortunately, this problem is less today than ten years ago, when physicians prescribed Valium for anyone complaining of nervousness. Because doctors now realize that drugs like Valium relieve anxiety only for a short period, they are prescribed less often than in the past. Yet I often see patients whose doctors prescribed Valium years earlier and who are still taking the medicine because their doctors are afraid to "rock the boat." Although Valium is a sedative, the sleep it produces is not normal, and you can awaken unrefreshed. Unless you are a heavy drinker, you can stop or cut down on alcohol by yourself; but eliminating drugs like Valium often requires help from a doctor.

Fatigue and Excess Weight

Overweight is another cause of fatigue that you can change. Being overweight means that you are carrying an excessive amount of fat on your frame. Since body weight is the sum of the weight of your skeletal frame, your muscles, your organs, and your fat, charts that give the range of weight for any particular age are not very helpful in determining whether any one individual is overweight. For example, such a chart would say that a 5'5" male weighing 200 pounds was overweight; but if he were a weightlifter, one would immediately see that he was not overweight and that his additional weight was in the form of muscle. One reasonable way of determining if you are overweight is the pinch test. Extend one arm and pinch the flesh on its underside halfway between your shoulder and your elbow. Since the skin and underlying tissues are quite thin, you will be pinching mostly fat. If you pinch more than one inch of fat, then you are probably overweight. Although you probably have a reasonably good sense of whether you are overweight, a visit to your doctor will let you know if you are right. The doctor will evaluate your body size and determine if you have excess fat. If so, it may explain your fatigue.

Fatigue and overweight go hand in hand for at least two reasons: first, the extra weight requires extra work to move; and second, the extra weight can block the air passages during sleep and lead to sleep apnea. If you are overweight and fatigued, losing weight should be your first treatment. There are many self-help books as well as groups like Weight Watchers whose purpose is to help you lose weight. Although a doctor's help is not essential for someone 20 pounds overweight, you might consider asking your doctor to devise a weight-loss program tailored for you. Besides advising you on the specifics of a diet, your doctor may prescribe an appetite suppressant. In the past, no medicine had been shown to specifically produce weight loss; Redux was the first such medicine. Unfortunately, Redux was withdrawn from the market because of serious adverse effects to the heart. Other similar drugs that should not share this toxicity are awaiting FDA approval. The three-pronged approach—diet, medication, and exercise—requires a real commitment from you, but if you make that commitment you will be rewarded. You will shed the weight, pound after pound.

The Architecture of a Night's Sleep

Finally, your fatigue may result from poor sleep or insomnia. For normal people, sleep comes soon after their lights are turned off and their head hits the pillow. Sleep has two basic forms: that occurring with rapid eye movements (REM sleep) and that occurring in the absence of rapid eye movements (non-REM sleep). When a healthy person falls asleep, the sleep becomes progressively deeper until about ninety minutes later, sleep lightens and becomes REM sleep. Whereas an individual might move about during the first part of sleep, motion stops when REM sleep begins. Instead of the body, the eyes move quickly back and forth. It is during this sleep period that dreams occur. Although the biological rhythm of REM sleep is such that it recurs on average every ninety minutes, it does occur more often at the end of a night than at the beginning. In contrast, the deepest non-REM sleep occurs in the first third of the sleep period.

Disruption of this normal pattern of sleep leads, as you might expect, to sleepiness and fatigue. Studies of patients awaiting surgery have found a preoperative reduction in deep sleep due to anticipation; this reduction can lead to the sensation of low energy. If anxiety is a chronic problem, the individual may undergo many brief periods of awakening, or an actual decrease in the total amount of deep sleep. Such repeated interruption of sleep may lead to daytime sleepiness.

Sleep Studies

If you experience extreme daytime fatigue without explanation, you will need a sleep study. Technical advances permit the sleep study in some cases to be done in the privacy of your own home. To be able to evaluate all causes of sleep disturbances, however, requires a night in a sleep lab. The results of such a study are often definitive in arriving at a diagnosis, and satisfactory medical treatments exist for the principal sleep disorders, sleep apnea and restless legs.

When neither of these diagnoses applies, yet the sleep study reveals insomnia or disturbed sleep, the sleep expert will begin to question your sleep habits. One can develop inappropriate sleep habits in much the same way that one can develop poor habits in other aspects of life. Because habits are slow to develop, you probably will not realize that they are the reason for your fatigue. One such habit is using one's bed as a desk or a reading chair. The connection between bed and sleep gets lost, and it becomes difficult for some people to fall asleep in their bed. Another habit is staying in bed if you cannot fall asleep. As a result, bed becomes mentally linked with sleeplessness. To cope with this problem, you *must* get out of bed and go to another room, where you should read or watch television until you are sleepy; then it is time to return to bed.

Although these habits are not difficult to break, recognizing the problem often requires the help of a professional expert in sleep. For the person with extreme daytime sleepiness, a sleep study will often produce positive results.

Treatments for Insomnia

The sleep expert first checks with you to be sure that you have eliminated excess stimulants from your diet—especially from noon on. Some common medicines have stimulants of which you may be unaware: the inhalants used by asthmatics to stop their wheezing, nose drops to clear a stuffed nose, and weight loss remedies. While each of these medicines certainly does what it is supposed to do, all share the side effect of being a stimulant that can certainly disturb sleep.

The next two steps have to do with your sleep habits. My father has trouble sleeping at night, but he naps regularly every day. Obviously daytime naps are going to interfere with normal nighttime sleep. You will have to work to stay awake during several days so that you will be able to sleep at night. The other thing to examine is the time you go to bed. It has to be standard, say eleven o'clock each night. If one night it is ten o'clock and another night one in the morning, that will make it harder for you to enjoy normal sleep each night.

Melatonin and Other Supplements

Our knowledge of what produces insomnia is still primitive. One substance that seems to play a role is melatonin, a hormone produced by the pineal gland in the brain. Originally, the function of melatonin was thought to pertain to skin color, but recent information points to a role in sleep and wakefulness. Scientific reports beginning to appear in the literature indicate that people with abnormal sleep patterns have abnormal patterns of melatonin secretion, and that small doses of melatonin may reduce sleeplessness.[1] Melatonin is currently available in health food stores as a dietary supplement. In that form it is not regulated, so problems of dosage exist. Melatonin disappears quickly from the bloodstream, so even though it may be effective in helping you fall asleep, its effect may wear off so that you wake up a few hours later. Drug companies are working to develop longer-lasting forms.

Another question relates to purity. Richard Wurtman, a physician and scientist at the Massachusetts Institute of Technology, tested six preparations available in health food stores. Only two proved to be pure, and the dosage was often not what the manufacturer indicated. Wurtman believes that the dose indicated on the package, 3 milligrams per pill, is far too high. He has done research with a tenth of that dose and has found it effective in inducing sleep. He feels the usual dosage may actually induce insomnia or produce a hangover. Thus melatonin is worth a try, but at reduced dosage. The Wurtman dose—somewhere between 0.3 milligram and 1 milligram of pure melatonin—may be available soon by prescription. If you do not find it, you could try the 3-milligram size most often sold in health food stores, but start with a quarter of a pill per night. (You will need to buy a pill splitter, because these pills can crumble in your hands if you try to split them.) The lower the dose, the less likelihood that it will produce side effects. Just because a product occurs naturally or within the body does not mean that taking it as a drug eliminates the risk that it may produce some toxicity.

The experience with tryptophan suggests that this matter should not be taken lightly. Tryptophan is one of the building blocks of food proteins and was shown early on to improve sleep. Since it was available in health food stores, people took it on their own for problems with sleep. By the late 1980s, nearly all the tryptophan that was made came from one source in Japan. Unfortunately the tryptophan somehow became contaminated, producing an illness characterized by severe and long-lasting pain in the muscles. Because of this problem of manufacture, tryptophan is no longer available to the public. However both it and its metabolite, 5-hydroxy-tryptophan, are available by prescription from a few mail-order pharmacies. Since the metabolite is closer to serotonin, the substance that actually causes sleep, it is reasonable to consider trying it—after discussion with your doctor. Many physicians hope that substances like melatonin and tryptophan will come under the regulatory supervision of the federal government. Should that occur, the consumer will have less freedom to self-medicate, but will be protected with regard to purity, dose, and—most important of all—efficacy.

Antihistamines as Sleep Aids

One drug that remains available over the counter is the antihistamine benadryl. Antihistamines are usually prescribed for itchiness, rashes, and runny or stuffed nose. Many patients were unable to take benadryl, the original antihistamine, because it produces extreme sleepiness. Today's new antihistamines no longer produce sleepiness, but the old standby is still available for people with insomnia.

The problem with benadryl is the kind of sleep it produces. For some people it works very well, while for others it produces a sort of twilight sleep where one is neither awake nor asleep. The drug has a different effect on the pattern of sleep from person to person. When effective, it regularizes the pattern of sleep and prevents the frequent microawakenings that can result from anxiety. In other words, the drug has then successfully treated the sleep disturbance. But when twilight sleep is the result, the drug has made the sleep pattern even more abnormal, resulting in even more fatigue.

Low-Dose Antidepressants
The other medicines used to treat insomnia are drugs that in high doses act as antidepressants, with the side effect of producing sleepiness. Interestingly, while their antidepressant effect disappears at lower doses, they still can produce sleep at these reduced doses. Thus, doctors can treat people with insomnia by prescribing low doses of sedating antidepressants such as Elavil, Sinequan, and Desyrel.

One class of drugs being used less and less is the sedatives: barbiturates sold as Nembutal, Seconal, or Luminal; chloral hydrate sold as Noctec; glutethimide sold as Doriden; and so on. These drugs had three major problems: relatively low doses could be lethal, they produced an abnormal and therefore often nonrestful sleep, and they were addicting. The same sorts of problems exist with the less dangerous class of drugs characterized by Valium. An additional problem of taking this drug and its cousins Ativan, Restoril, and Halcion is that the sleep-enhancing effect wears off. The drug works like a charm for a few weeks, then loses its effectiveness. The result can be a habit that is difficult to break. An individual can be given this medicine to help reduce insomnia caused by some recent stress and to relieve the stress that comes from sleeplessness. The medicine works and the patient sleeps; at the same time the problem either disappears or becomes less intense. But taking the pill and falling asleep become associated in the person's mind, so when the patient skips the pill, he or she cannot sleep. Furthermore, stopping the pills produces a mild withdrawal state characterized by anxiety and sleeplessness. Thus the treatment can become its own illness. The problem is much less serious for those who do not need to take the medicine every night. Taken two or three times a week, the sedating effect usually remains and the problems are minimal.

New Alternatives

For today's patients with insomnia, these sedatives are no longer the first line of treatment should prescription drugs be necessary. Low doses of antidepressants, which carry sedation as a side effect, are the better alternative. Another option, a new medicine called Ambien, is a sedative with less of a down side than the Valium-type medicines— much less of a hung-over or woozy feeling the morning after taking it.[7] Like any other sedative, it can produce some nervousness and increased sleep problems if it is halted abruptly. If the drug disagrees with you or seems to be losing its effectiveness, you will need to consult your doctor before stopping it, especially if you have used it for more than a few weeks. Ambien works best if taken on an empty stomach, so the appropriate time is a half-hour before sleep is desired. The medicine is known to be effective in chronic insomnia for over a month; whether it remains effective for longer periods is not currently known. But it is a "best bet" for relieving insomnia without the side effects of the other sleep inducers.

7 ℂ The Role of Exercise in Reducing Stress

Probably the most common cause of fatigue is stress, whether you recognize it or not. One form is very easy to recognize—you are suddenly confronted with something that frightens or upsets you. But the small annoyances of everyday life—someone cutting into the line in front of you, a red light when you are a bit late, seeing someone you would rather not see—these minor stresses often produce fatigue because they require an effort on your part to push beyond them. If you are in a situation or a job where you face many of these minor stresses, you may feel exhausted at the end of the day.

Fatigue and effort seem totally incompatible; but, surprisingly, effort in the form of aerobic exercise relieves the fatigue of stress. Exactly how exercise works is unclear, but feelings of stress, anxiety, and fatigue can disappear following exercise.[1] The problem with prescribing exercise as a treatment of fatigue is that exercise is hard to start. Physical fitness builds on the level of fitness you currently have. So if your fitness level is low, moving it up a notch is difficult. If, on the other hand, you are not sedentary and have some degree of fitness already, it is easier to become more fit.

The issues are the same for someone who has fatigue due to an illness like chronic fatigue syndrome except that for such a person it is even harder to get started. The critical thing to remember is that regardless of your condition or illness, resting or staying in bed reduces your fitness level. In fact, that is precisely what bedrest is used to do in studies of the effects of life in space. Inactivity and/or bedrest produces the same drop in fitness that life in space produces, so it is a handy tool for developing treatments to maintain fitness in space. If you are healthy but rest a lot, are aged and frail and thus limited in your ability to get around, or have any kind of chronic illness that requires bedrest, you can be sure that some of the fatigue you experience is due to your lack of fitness. Your body recognizes the minimal effort needed to do your normal daily activities as exercise, and since your fitness level is low, the effort—although minimal—produces more fatigue.

This formula of fitness as hard to start and becoming easier to maintain and even improve is responsible for most people's quitting fitness programs. In the United States incredible amounts of money are spent on pieces of fitness equipment for the home, which often end up as horizontal filing cabinets for clothes, papers, and items not to be misplaced. The major issue is getting started, and doing that costs nothing.

The First Steps

The first step is to do something physical, to get away from the bed and the easy chair. Whether you are basically well or have some sort of fatiguing illness, touch base with your doctor to determine what you can do. My own exercise prescription usually is that a person walk, and I try to tailor the prescription to the individual. For some, a start could be walking to the corner to mail a letter; for others, walking around a mall and window shopping—if only for five minutes. Rarely, for very sick patients with CFS, I recommend that they go to a toning center. There the machines move you rather than your moving the machines, but again it is a first step. If successful, it will allow you to start walking later. If you prefer to use a treadmill (either at home or at a fitness center), that is fine, but you must start slowly. That means strolling at a slow pace—0.5 to 1.5 miles per hour.

The point to remember is that there is *no rush* to improve your fitness. In fact, if you push too hard or too fast, the result could be unpleasant. That is what makes people abandon their fitness machines and their New Year's resolutions to improve their state of fitness. If you are sedentary, it has taken months, perhaps years, for you to reach your current level of low fitness. If you have an illness that requires resting or being in bed, your fitness level will be even lower. So the *gradual approach,* starting with very mild exercise, must be the rule.

Pacing yourself is not a trivial task, especially for goal-oriented, time-conscious people. Still, to do so is critical if you are to succeed in improving your fitness. If your problem is just fatigue, the minimum time between changes in amount of exercise should be one week, assuming that you exercise three times per week; it should be longer if you are sick with an illness like chronic fatigue syndrome. And increases should be kept modest: a trial of walking for those who could do no exercise at all and have tried the toning-table route; an increase in walking time from five to seven minutes for people who were able to exercise. Remember that you are looking for an ability to do increased work without making yourself feel more fatigued or sick.

Obviously, exercise will be fatiguing. Slowly but surely, though, the fatigue that is produced will lessen, as will feelings of anxiety or stress. One important caveat: plan to do your exercising at least four hours before bedtime. As your exercise time increases, the result will be a drop in fatigue. So if you exercise shortly before bedtime, you may have more of a problem falling asleep. Several hours following exercise, a rebound of fatigue often occurs, and this will help with your sleep. Because of this pattern, exercise is an important part of the treatment of fatigue.

CFS and Exercise

Some of you may be saying that this is all well and good for someone who has simple fatigue, but what about a person with chronic fatigue syndrome? Arguments rage over whether patients with severe and chronic fatigue should exercise or not. One of the elements that adds to the confusion is that a common complaint of CFS patients is that exertion, even when quite mild, produces a flarcup of their symptoms. The problem is the interplay between the illness and the drop in fitness that inactivity brings. Certainly if you are in the phase of the illness where you have fever and extreme malaise that keeps you in bed, you should not consider exercise. The timing would make as much sense as exercising while you have the flu. But many of my patients experience different phases in their CFS. For instance, it is not at all uncommon for the fever and sore throat to go away. Even if these do not disappear, many patients find that they can spend a substantial period of time out of bed. They may still be disabled and unable to work because of their symptoms, but they will be able to exercise—at least a little.

Stress Testing

We have done research on twenty-two CFS patients of this sort.[2] We did actual exercise stress testing, consisting of walking at a fast rate until the patients could not walk further. We compared these results to those of healthy people who did not exercise regularly. Not surprisingly, the CFS group (who all said that their activity level was substantially reduced compared to levels before their illness) were less fit than the healthy group. However, the difference was relatively small. Had we found a comparison group of people who were extremely sedentary, we suspect we would not have found any difference between the groups.

This extreme exercise challenge produced serious flareups in only a few patients. But the exercise did have a measurable negative effect on the CFS patients' ability to do *mental* work after the stress test. A check with our patients and with our healthy comparison subjects about their fatigue following the stress test revealed that the healthy people felt less fatigue. The patients' fatigue did get worse, but not strikingly so. That surprised us, because a common complaint of the CFS patient is that even mild exercise produces a worsening of overall condition and fatigues them sufficiently that they often have to go to bed. It is possible that the short burst of high-intensity exertion demanded in our stress test is not the type of exertion that produces this pattern of worsening. Learning exactly what kind of exertion produces symptom flareups will take research. Since a maximal stress test did not produce serious flareups of illness, we believe that less intensive physical exertion will not do so either. That is why we are beginning to prescribe gentle fitness training for patients with CFS.

Fitness Training for CFS

The exertion we induced was of an experimental nature and is not what we would suggest to a patient. All the same, it makes the point that fitness training is a possibility for patients with severe fatigue. Indeed, several groups have shown that fitness training makes fibromyalgia patients feel better;[3] since patients with fibromyalgia plus fatigue probably have CFS, these studies augur well for the CFS patient. In fact, my colleagues in our rehabilitation department have done fitness training on nearly a hundred CFS patients with encouraging results. Furthermore, a recent Australian study reported the results of a treatment trial of gentle conditioning in CFS and concluded that it is not only effective but that it continues to reduce CFS symptoms many months later.[4] The totality of these experiences tells us that fitness training, monitored by a trained physical therapist and individually tailored for the patient, should be part of the management of CFS for appropriate patients.

The goal of the exercise regimen depends on the person. If you have been unable to walk at all, five minutes of walking is a major achievement. But I try to ask everyone to aim for twenty minutes of walking at a quick pace. If a person can attain this goal, then I raise it to thirty minutes at the same quick pace. Achievement of the twenty-minute goal of course depends on the person. If you are in good health but have been extremely sedentary, you can attain this goal in about a month, but it will take much longer if you have a fatiguing illness such as CFS. And disappointments will come. For the CFS patient, there is often a narrow line between being able to exercise at all and the worsening of symptoms that too much exercise brings. Indeed, I have a few male CFS patients who are fine as long as they can remain sedentary. These patients are the exception: they can work and have a normal life as long as they can live a very tranquil life with no physical demands. If they have to meet even as mild a demand as walking a long distance from office to car, by the time they reach the car they begin to feel feverish and achy. Obviously the kind of exercise that I am recommending here will not work for them.

Tai Chi

Two other forms of exercise may be helpful in combating fatigue. The first is a very gentle muscular conditioning, used for millennia in China, called tai chi. It consists of a series of exercises that are easy to perform and can be done daily. I have been impressed that some of my sickest CFS patients are able to do the tai chi exercises, and they report less fatigue and pain thereafter. Although we know nothing of how such exercise works, it certainly must counteract the biological effects of inactivity. One can learn the exercises either at one of the many courses on tai chi taught at local colleges or at a fitness center.

Another alternative is to buy a videotape that demonstrates the exercises. (One of these is performed by the actor David Carradine and costs $19.95; to order, call 1-800-972-5800.)

Kundalini Yoga

Our knowledge about the final form of exercise that I want to mention is even more rudimentary, but it is logical that it might be helpful in the treatment of fatigue. The system of exercises called kundalini yoga is more diverse and usually more active than the stretching and static posture form of hatha yoga that is more common in the United States. Kundalini yoga uses various combinations of patterns of breathing and muscular exertion. Breathing as regularly as a metronome has a major influence on the heart. If you check the pulse in your neck or wrist while you breathe slowly and regularly, you will feel your pulse rate increase while you breathe in and decrease while you breathe out.

Regular breathing has this effect on the heart via a nerve called the vagus. When firing of the vagus nerve diminishes, heart rate increases; when firing increases, heart rate slows. In addition to these effects on the heart, the vagus nerve plays an important role in hastening digestion. Slowing of the heart and turning on digestive processes are what happens in the abscence of stress; when stress exists, vagal firing stops, and heart rate increases while digestion stops. Thus one way of viewing the vagus is as a nerve whose function it is to combat arousal or stress. We have learned that it works at subnormal levels in CFS.[5] This fact may explain, at least in part, why the CFS patient is so often stress sensitive.

Although biological knowledge of the effects of breathing and muscular tension is limited, the fact that these exercises have been practiced for millennia in India suggests that they may have therapeutic effects, especially in relieving anxiety and stress. In fact, a recent study supports the idea that breathing at slow regular rates may achieve this goal.[6] The researchers told volunteers that they would receive an unpleasant electric shock. The shock was never given, but the researchers monitored vagal activity during the period of anticipation. It decreased when volunteers breathed spontaneously or when they breathed at rapid metronomic rates; such a decrease would be expected during stress. The decrease was not found when the volunteers breathed at regular slow rates.

In addition to the possible stress-relieving effects of paced breathing, these sorts of breathing exercises may be specifically useful for the CFS patient by increasing the function of their vagus nerves. (You can get access to North American or international teachers of this form of yoga—kundalini yoga, as taught by Yogi Bhajan—by calling the following U.S. phone number: 310-552-3416.)

One U.S. practitioner, researcher, and teacher, David Shannahoff-Khalsa, can be reached by mail at the Institute for Nonlinear Science, University of California, 9500 Gillman Drive, La Jolla, CA 92093-0402. He has published on yogic techniques[7] and suggests the two given below to counteract stress and to relieve fatigue.

Method 1. Sit and maintain a straight spine. Relax the arms and place your hands in your lap. Focus your eyes on the tip of your nose. (You cannot see the end, just the sides of the nose.) Open your mouth as wide as possible, slightly stressing the temporal-mandibular joint; touch the tip of your tongue to the upper palate, where it is hard and smooth. Breathe continuously through the nose only, while making the respiration slow and deep. Concentrate on the sound of your breathing. Listen to it as you inhale and exhale. Set a kitchen timer, and the first time you do this exercise do not exceed three minutes. Do it daily, and very gradually (a couple of minutes per week) increase your time to a maximum of twenty minutes.

Method 2. Not to be done if you are pregnant or have high blood pressure. Sit as above and again look toward the tip of your nose. Try to pull your nose toward your upper lip by actually pulling your upper lip down over the front teeth by using the muscles in the upper lip.

Leaving the mouth open during the exercise helps you do this. There are three stages to this exercise. (1) Inhale deeply while raising your hands above your head, then tightly clench your fists and tense your forearms and slowly pull your fists down toward your abdomen. (2) Hold your breath and maintain the tension in your fists and forearms. Bring your shoulders up toward your ears while tightly tensing your shoulders and neck muscles as you raise them. (3) Exhale and relax the muscles. Between each repetition keep the eyes focused on the tip of the nose and the upper lip pulled down. Repeat this entire exercise six times.

It would be reasonable to try these exercises any time you are feeling stressed or tense or want to feel calm. It is best not to try them after meals while the stomach is in action, but a few hours later—before bedtime—might help with insomnia. As a sign of the effectiveness of these exercises, look for improved sleep and less tension within three weeks of starting. As with all prescriptions, I recommend trying them for up to six weeks. Then if you are not convinced that anything is happening, stop and compare how you felt while doing the exercises to how you feel after you stopped.

8 ⟨ Identifying and Coping with Stress

The next two chapters aim to teach you how to identify stress and how to deal with it. Stress management is the cottage industry of the 1990s. Everywhere one looks there are courses, work-site programs, self-help books, videos, and audiocassettes on how to manage stress. This chapter will introduce the ideas behind stress management. For some readers, the thought of seeking help to manage your stress level will make a lot of sense; others may tell themselves, "no way." Those in the latter category have a lot in common with many others who claim to have no use for professional help for any nonphysical problem—especially one that requires coping with the problems of everyday life. But reading this chapter will show you how simple these techniques are. Even if you still do not want professional help to improve your ability to cope with the stresses in your life, you may elect to try these techniques on your own.

Identifying Stress in Yourself
You cannot start to manage your stress if you cannot identify it in yourself. Stress takes many different forms, which vary from person to person. Without spending the time to learn your own personal

response to stressful situations, you may not recognize when you are under stress and will not be able to intervene in stressful situations. One thing about stress is the same for everyone: it causes them to burn energy, so it results in fatigue. Thus anything that will help to stop stress will reduce fatigue.

The easiest way to recognize stress in yourself is first to recognize it in others. A number of common situations elicit stress in most people and should be your primary targets for observation and learning. These are usually situations in which unanticipated delays occur (having to wait in line at the supermarket checkout counter or at the bank) or where deadlines exist (having to change planes quickly in an unfamiliar airport). Or an unanticipated delay and a deadline can exist at the same time in a traffic jam on your way to the airport to catch a plane.

Different people react differently to stressful situations. In a traffic jam, an easily irritated person may explode, start swearing, slam his fist on the steering wheel, and honk even though none of these reactions will help. In contrast, the next car may hold a nervous sort, who may chew his nails, need a cigarette, or keep checking his watch as each minute passes. Observe the wide variety of reactions people have in such situations. Look for behavioral symptoms such as fidgeting or a tense, upset look on the face. Look for emotional symptoms such as expressions of worry, fear, or surprising irritability.

Now that you have some idea of what stress does to others, begin evaluating what it does to you. It makes sense to study yourself in situations that are commonly stress producing. When you notice that you are feeling tense or irritated, ask yourself, "Is something bothering me? What has triggered this reaction?" An obvious answer is that it may be stress. Appreciating stress in yourself will give you clues about identifying symptoms that the person under stress feels but does not necessarily show. Watch for behavioral symptoms, which include muscle tightness or aching. Check for emotional symptoms, which include feelings of restlessness, tension, worry, or the presence of anxious thoughts. This is the time to look within yourself to see some of the other ways stress can affect you.

Connections between Brain and Bodily Organs

Stress turns on the connections between your brain and your heart, muscles, digestive system, or urinary bladder. I previously made the point that it also turns off such connections as vagal nerve activity. All these changes may make you aware of your heart beating faster or less regularly than usual; you may develop a headache or back spasm; you may develop a "nervous stomach," which may produce a stomach-ache, nausea, vomiting, or a sudden attack of diarrhea; or you may develop a "nervous bladder," which shows itself as the need to urinate frequently or the feeling that unless you get to the bathroom quickly you will wet yourself. Symptoms like these can be a real problem when you are in a closed car stuck in traffic on your way to the airport.

Although stress varies greatly from person to person, the pattern of symptoms that it produces in any individual remains quite constant from day to day. If you recognize in yourself muscle tension, feelings of anxiety, and a nervous bladder at times of stress, your body understands these symptoms: you are under stress.

Chronic Stress

All of the examples thus far have to do with acute stress—your body's response to the aggravation of an incident that happens suddenly and unexpectedly. But stress can be of long duration also, and it is this form that has major biological and psychological consequences, most often evident in the form of fatigue and worry. So you need to examine also your body's response to chronic stress.

Look for the same manifestations as in acute stress, but recognize that there will be more of them and they will have longer-term consequences. Worrying about the security of your job or an important task lasting several days or weeks can produce a pattern of weekday tension headaches—a tight band-like pain in the back of the neck that worsens as the day goes on. The effects of stress can carry over into sleep to produce tooth grinding, which translates into a sore jaw during the day. Chronic stress can also change the way you deal with people. If it makes you irritable, you will find yourself being stand-offish or having a chip on your shoulder (getting angry with innocent telephone operators who put you on hold); but it can also make you more "people hungry" to provide a way to relax and escape the stress. Finally, chronic stress can change your appetites—for food, for tobacco, for sex. You may find yourself eating more or less, with proportional changes in your weight, or you may find yourself smoking more, or starting to smoke again after you had successfully quit. And you may notice a marked loss of interest in sex.

Your Stress Buttons

With this attention to people around you and finally to yourself, you should be able to identify your own particular stress response. The next step in your personal stress management program is to figure out which situations produce this stress response. Everyone has his or her own set of buttons that reliably produce the stress state when pushed. Some of these buttons (our traffic jam, for instance) are widely shared. But you will have your specific buttons: they could be contact with a relative, a problem at work, a misunderstanding with a child. The formula is always the same, but the solution varies from person to person. If you can identify your own stress triggers, that is the critical next step in managing your stress.

As you begin to identify those situations that stress you, you will be able to start coping with them more effectively. To do this, you have to divide the situations that produce stress in you into two groups, situations you can alter or modify and those you cannot. Then you can pursue two tactics to manage the stressors in your life: do whatever is necessary to change a situation that puts you under stress, and when this is not possible, deal with the emotional consequences of being in that kind of a stressful situation.

Removing Sources of Stress

The sorts of situations a person will accept without making any effort to change are sometimes amazing. For if you are in a situation that chronically puts you under stress, "change" is the key word. If you can change the situation, the stress will disappear. So you have to take action to remove the sources of stress. You do this by looking at the stressful situation as you would a puzzle. If your landlord is hassling you, think through what you can do to make him stop; if that does not work, you have to consider moving. If you have CFS and you find yourself stressed by family members who refuse to believe that you are sick, give them literature on CFS or ask your doctor to speak with them about the nature of your illness. A person's illness can also be magnified by one's refusal to accept the problem. It happens frequently with CFS. Patients become frustrated because their lives have changed, and instead of accepting this fact, they fight it and try to live as they did previously. The energy expended is huge, and the results of the effort are often the opposite of those desired, in that symptoms often get worse. By realizing you are in this vicious circle, you can step back from the heat and give recovery a chance.

One situation that is often very stressful occurs when you need to do more things than you have time to do. Particularly when you are sick, your illness reduces the time you have available for *any* activities, and your fatigue limits your ability to use the time that is available. Basically, thinking through and organizing how you spend your day, whether you are healthy or ill, gains you more time.

Let's look at healthy people first: they often organize their time to do the tasks that are quick and easy. They make quick phone calls, run easy errands, make photocopies. They like to scratch things off their lists. If they do something not on their list, they sometimes write it down so that they can scratch it off. They put off the bigger, important jobs they really need to do. They say to themselves, "I've got to get these other things out of the way first." The problem is that days can go by and that important task does not get done. At the end of the day, they realize they still haven't got the real work done, and they feel stressed.

Managing Time Better

You—all of us—can do a better job of managing time. You need to take a few moments at the end or the beginning of each day to decide what has to be done the next day. Make a list. Then divide that list into A, B, and C priorities. A is for the items that are the most important and need to be started or finished, B items are important but can wait, and C items are either not so important or can wait. Two things about this list will amaze you. First, you will see that you are probably spending the bulk of your time on tasks that you rate as C or B in importance; and, second, you may find that the things on your A list alone add up to more hours than you have available that day. Prioritize everything on the A list. Start the day with the A list's top priority. If it is a big job, do only the first step. Work at the A list top priority for about a half-hour and then take a break.

Pay attention to how you feel. Many people feel a real sense of accomplishment and relief. They say, "I finally got it started" or "It doesn't seem so big and impossible to do." While on your break, do a top-priority task from the B list, something that is quick and easy. Go ahead and scratch it off the list. You've earned the right! Now, consider spending another half-hour on the A list. Later, as the day comes to a close, give yourself a few minutes to plan tomorrow. If you have to bring work home in the evening, resist the temptation to bring more than you can possibly do. Think about making more general lists of A's, B's, and C's for the week. These lists will help you to say no. Staying within the bounds of reality will stop people from getting angry at you for having said yes but having done nothing. The result of effective time management is that you have more time to relax and you burn less energy. Both result in less fatigue.

Managing time is as much a problem for the sick as it is for the well. When the problem is pointed out to them, patients seem to do better than healthy people, because their day is shorter: the limitations imposed upon them by illness and their ability to perform are similarly reduced by the available resources. CFS is a good example. Patients learn they only have so much energy to expend in one day, so they rapidly learn to invest their energy carefully to do the one task that is most important for them that day. Having limitations makes it imperative to say no. Because patients are forced to learn effective time management techniques, they seem to do better managing their time after they recover. In this sense, illness helps one to restructure one's life.

Reducing the Emotional Stress Response

The second part of coping with stress has to do with reducing one's emotional response to stressful situations, particularly to situations that cannot be changed. By emotional response, I mean the fast heart rate, the nausea, and the muscle tightness that come with stress. One turns to emotion-based coping when it is either impossible or impractical to try to change the stress-provoking situation. Perhaps the simplest way is to use imagery.

Imagination and Imagery

Imagine yourself in a situation that you find relaxing. It might be a favorite vacation spot or your favorite room at home. It might be listening to soothing music. Each person can create the "perfect" image to use. Since many people choose the same sort of relaxing images, it is not surprising to know of the existence of audiocassettes describing many of these images. You can find them in any large store that sells tapes or CDs. Usually it is helpful to use these relaxation tapes as an aid.

First, stretch out in a place where you can be comfortable and will not be disturbed. Close your eyes and relax, and while the tape unwinds, let your mind create the scene for yourself. Fill in all the details. If it's a beach scene, feel the warm sun, hear the sea gulls and the waves. If it's at a mountain stream, smell the fresh air, listen to the water and the wind in the trees rustling the leaves, hear the song of a distant bird. Stay in the scene for ten minutes or so. If the imagery has worked, you should feel relaxed and tranquil, with none of the speeding, anxious thoughts you experienced just minutes before. Remember too that when relaxation works, it is a fine tool to combat insomnia. Become comfortable with the technique and then try it before bedtime. You may be astounded at how well imagery relaxes you.

Progressive Muscle Relaxation

The second relaxation technique is called progressive muscle relaxation (PMR), which can also be helped by audiocassettes designed specifically to achieve this form of relaxation. Progressive muscular relaxation helps you attain by yourself what imagery aims to produce. Imagery takes your mind off the events that are producing the symptoms of stress in your body. Developed in the 1930s, PMR helps you to learn the feelings of muscular tension that are frequently produced in stressful situations, and to learn the feelings of relaxation that occur in pleasant situations. Once you know these feelings, you can learn how to turn them on and off. You then have a powerful tool to combat muscle tension whenever stress arises, as well as one to ensure relaxation and normal sleep at the end of a busy day. By learning how to relax your muscles, you will combat fatigue, stress, and their offspring—anxiety and depression.

Succeeding at PMR requires your active participation. As in learning any other new skill—be it playing the piano or skiing—you must first pay attention, then practice. The technique used to produce relaxation requires you to tense certain muscles on command. The result is that you can feel maximal muscle tension. Eventually you will be able to compare the degree of muscle tension in your body with what is maximal. It is important to understand that every person in a state of wakefulness has some degree of muscular tension; it is what permits you to move from one place to another, to do things during your waking day. Frequently, however, stress turns up your muscle tension with the inevitable consequence of fatigue. By knowing the feeling of your maximal muscle tension, your muscle tension at the end of a busy day, and the absence of muscle tension following relaxation, you will be able to judge your stress level and reduce it when needed.

To learn how to perform PMR, you will first maximally tense your muscles and then suddenly relax and release all the tension in the muscle. The procedure is very similar to the kundalini yoga exercise described in the last chapter. Here you do this tightening and relaxing of muscles in a progressive way, stepping through all the muscle groups of the body. Tension becomes a tool to help you feel what it is like to have relaxed muscles. Thus you will learn the difference between muscle tension and muscle relaxation, and will be able to produce either state in your body at will.

The following are the sixteen muscle groups to tense and the way to achieve tension in those groups.

1. Right hand and forearm: make a fist.

2. Right biceps: push elbow down against chair or floor.

3. Left hand and forearm: make a fist.

4. Left biceps: push elbow down against chair or floor.

5. Forehead: lift eyebrows as high as possible.

6. Upper cheeks and nose: squint eyes and wrinkle nose.

7. Lower cheeks and jaw: bite hard and pull back corners of mouth.

8. Neck and throat: pull chin toward chest but do not let it touch chest.

9. Chest, shoulders, and upper back: pull shoulder blades together.

10. Abdomen: make stomach muscles hard.

11. Right thigh: press buttock into chair or floor.

12. Right calf: pull toes toward head.

13. Right foot: point and curl toes, turning foot inward.

14. Left thigh: press buttock into chair or floor.

15. Left calf: pull toes toward head.

16. Left foot: point and curl toes, turning foot inward.

Learning either or both of these techniques—emotion-based coping and progressive muscle relaxation—will give you powerful tools to use in your personal stress-management program.

9 ⟨ Help from a Coach or Consultant

Developing and following a personal stress-management program of the sort discussed in the last chapter requires self-discipline, an attribute not all of us possess. Some of you may benefit from help in managing your stress. Since stress management is a growth industry in this country, you will have no problem finding someone to help you. Classes in stress management are now given at the workplace, at community centers and hospitals, and at universities. The one advantage of going to an "expert" in stress management is that you can tell him or her what sort of help you need. I like to view such experts as coaches or consultants, who give you advice and help you make it work. The only problem with going to any particular coach is that any such expert will have his or her own specific approach to the problem of stress, and you will need to be comfortable with that approach.

It is important to understand that relaxation techniques are only one of several choices for stress management. Another very important technique requires your getting into a dialogue with the coach about why you are stressed and what can be done about it. The kind of training that allows someone to perform this service has broadened considerably in the last few years. The individual's background and training can be in medicine, psychology, social work, or even religion. The cost for a session with such a consultant decreases from physician to minister, but it is important to realize that the coach's degree has nothing to do with how good the individual is at the job. So my advice to people considering this approach is to find someone with a strong reputation and relatively low rates. What is important is whether you feel comfortable with the person.

Assistance with Emotion-Based Coping

In the last chapter I discussed how important it was to break down the sources of stress in your life into those that you can deal with to reduce or avoid and those that cannot be avoided and thus require emotional coping. For some of you, the guidelines and examples in Chapter 8 will be enough to get you started, but others of you will need help. Being able to step away to view yourself and your problems "objectively" is a skill that not everyone has. You may need the help of a coach.

If you have an illness such as AIDS or CFS, the coach will help you understand that you cannot do anything to erase the diagnosis. But coaches can give you some ideas on how to escape it, if for only a brief time. Some of the possibilities could include taking a vacation from your illness—a long weekend at an exotic place where you can escape the consequences of being sick—or joining a self-help or support group of people who suffer from the same condition. In addition to these temporary ways to reduce stress, they may use stress-reduction techniques to help you cope more effectively. The net result of your visits to the coach will be to reduce your stress level, which will immediately reduce your physical symptoms.

For those of you who are not ill, it is important to remember that these stress-reducing techniques do not simply help people whose stress is magnified by disease. Unfortunately, some social situations produce the same effect as these chronic incurable diseases. I know several couples where the partners cannot stand each other but are locked together for financial reasons. Let's suppose that you are in this situation—which may seem as inescapable for you as AIDS. Yet your options for coping with such an "incurable" problem are a lot broader than they are if you have cancer. You can escape for a long weekend, you can visit a friend once a week, you can try to arrange your schedule so that you see little of your partner.

In contrast to situations that are not changeable are other stressful situations that result from problems that can be handled, to a greater or lesser degree. Depending on who you are, you may or may not be able to find solutions. In most instances it is worthwhile to seek information and advice as the first step in problem solving. Here again, a stress-management expert may be helpful, as well as others who have particular skills in this area.

Examples and Solutions

Let us look at some examples of problems and ways to solve them. If you have trouble talking to your boss, consider a class in communications. If you have trouble talking to your partner, couples counseling may be the solution. If you are having trouble making ends meet, consider seeing a financial advisor. If your doctor does not seem to understand your concerns, talk to the nurse or consider finding a new doctor.

A coach will help you first to identify the feeling of stress. He (or she) may do that by asking you about situations that make you nervous or worried, and then ask you to imagine that you are in such a situation. Result: dry mouth, racing heart, and the need to urinate. Instead of learning about stress by observing other people, the coach helps you understand it in yourself. It is astonishing what a second person can see through the eyes of the first. Having done that, he can help you see the things in your life that could be causing the stress.

Usually these "fixes" take the form of relatively small changes—adjusting your schedule so you do not see every day the person who makes your blood boil; or making minor alterations in your home or work environment.

Often, relatively straightforward solutions exist that will help you with these sorts of problems. One common way of dealing with stress is to bypass or ignore the problem. Unfortunately, that strategy frequently requires more effort than learning how to go from start to finish in the shortest, least painful way. The coach may see an easy way for you to change your way of reacting to allow you to go around the stress. A second simple solution might involve your seeking friends or family who will give you support in a stressful situation. Because you may be uncomfortable in burdening those nearest to you, a coach will first act as your source of support; he is there for you to unload on him. But the coach may also have ideas concerning those to whom you might turn in your circle of friends and family. Finally, the coach may help you become more assertive, to stand up for your rights. Sometimes turning the other cheek is not the correct solution.

Another area where you might need some help is time management. If you find that you cannot say no and seem to have more work than results at the end of the day, or seem to always have an excuse for being unable to get anything done, you will need help in the better use of your time. How to get such help depends on where you are. Many adult education programs give short courses on time management, as do local colleges; if these are not available in your area, you will find books on time management in the "self-help" section of your local bookstore or library.

Helping you see what you have missed is the easier part of the coach's work. Some people are much more stress sensitive than others because of their perception of how they fit within their personal and professional worlds. Based on who you are and how you feel about your fit, certain situations may produce an automatic but distorted response that expands minor stressful occurrences into huge problems. Here are some examples.

Go to a social event → Sit in the corner because no one will want to meet me.

Decide not to apply for a job that everyone says is tailor made for you → Why should I? I'll never succeed.

A co-worker takes advantage of you → I won't do anything but grin and bear it. No one will listen anyhow.

The Ellis Approach

These illogical mental leaps seem to occur on their own and are often followed by feelings of distress. Albert Ellis, a psychologist who developed much of this thinking, says that these feelings of distress stem from what he calls the philosophy of "Musturbation."[1] By this he means that people believe that they "must" or "must not" behave a certain way, or respond to a situation in a certain way, even if that behavior or response is at odds with what they really want.

Here the job of the coach is to make you grasp the concept of automatic negative thinking, so that you no longer think you "must" act out these thoughts, to personalize these concepts so that you can see your own automatic negative thoughts and what produces them, and understand how your reaction to events occurring around you alters your behavior, the way you feel about yourself, and the confidence with which you present yourself to others. The final step is to help you stop making these distortions and thus get out of a vicious cycle.

Aaron Beck, a pioneering physician who built on Ellis' approach to relieving stress, has written a book about it that is very readable; another book for the layperson was a best-seller when it was published.[2] Beck calls the technique cognitive restructuring; psychologists call it cognitive behavioral therapy. Its crucial lesson is that you can learn *not* to have these negative thoughts and you can exclude words like "should" and "must" from your mental vocabulary.

Examples of Automatic Thinking

It does not take long to learn whether or not you have these automatic but distorted responses and to see the circumstances that trigger them. Surprisingly, once you understand the buttons that seem to put you in the same stressful situation time and time again, you can quickly learn to avoid them. A coach can usually help you achieve these goals over a short period—several weeks to a month or two. To help you better understand the concept of automatic negative thinking, let me give you some examples of how such thinking can occur.

1. One rather common automatic reaction is jumping to conclusions based on too little information. The result can be a serious misinterpretation of the truth and the generation of serious stress. The process can happen in two ways. In the first, you think you know what other people are thinking about you and jump to conclusions without checking out that thinking. An example might be a social situation where you are introduced to someone who was having an active conversation with someone else earlier but who has little to say to you. You might conclude that this person is reacting negatively to you, when in fact, the person may be quite shy and previously was able to communicate actively because the other person was a close friend.

If you are by nature pessimistic and/or negative, you can reach the wrong conclusion in another way. Your negativity may make you feel that things will turn out badly for you. You don't question that belief; you automatically believe it, acting like a fortune teller who sees only misery in your future. Accepting these negative thoughts as fact is of course unrealistic.

2. Another set of problems comes from negativism. Some people

are just more negative than others. If you are one of these, automatic negative thinking will happen frequently unless you fight it. Something negative happens and you tell yourself that once it has happened, it will happen again and again. And if something positive happens to you, you tend to ignore it. For example, someone at work tells you that you are doing a good job and you write it off as simple politeness.

3. There is a situation I call the social paradox. You may feel very insecure about your relations with other people and believe that people do not care about you. However, when something unfortunate or annoying happens in a social context, you put the blame on yourself. Say you are planning to join a group of friends to go to the movies; someone cannot make it, so the plans are canceled. Instead of saying to yourself that these things happen, you tell yourself that the evening fell apart because people did not want to be with you. Although on the one hand you think no one notices you, on the other hand you think your presence is incredibly powerful in a negative sense.

4. A final example is the mountain out of the molehill syndrome and its opposite, the molehill out of the mountain. You think you performed poorly on a test and tell yourself that the professor and your friends will think you are an idiot. (This is also an example of your being the inaccurate fortune teller discussed in example 1.) I know one student who does this all the time: complains of poor performance on a test, worries about what people will think, and then finds an *A* on the test. This constitutes very poor fortune telling and making a mountain out of a molehill. Tied in is selling yourself short. Instead of learning that you are really an *A* student, you tell yourself you did an awful job on the test but the student assistant just let it slide by.

Techniques of Cognitive Restructuring

The important lesson derived from these examples of automatic negative thinking is that such thinking makes a person feel insecure, nervous, and stressed. The end point of this emotional outpouring of energy is fatigue. Although one's basic personality is highly resistant to change, a vulnerable negative person can learn to cope with and resist the tendency to have automatic negative thoughts. These thoughts can be changed: they occur in all of us, even the most positive and outgoing types. Breaking the links of automatic thinking in itself relieves stress and eases fatigue. It lets you concentrate on the positive elements of your life—which are often pleasant, relaxing, and nonstressful.

These techniques of cognitive restructuring play an important role in the treatment of CFS. As with AIDS or MS, no cure exists—but improvement is possible. Chapter 12 will be devoted to the medical treatment of CFS, but I must warn you in advance that no medical treatment has proved efficacious in more than one study. As I have indicated previously, a result—even a therapeutic one—is not valid unless a second group shows that it can obtain the same result. And no putative medical treatment of CFS has ever been replicated.

In contrast, two groups have now done controlled trials showing that cognitive restructuring greatly helps reduce CFS symptoms.[3] For patients who are afraid to become active, cognitive restructuring helps them see that the results of effort are not "awful" (to use the patients' term), although they may produce some worsening of symptoms for several days. The treatment offers the CFS patient new and effective coping mechanisms to confront the often self-defeating option of staying in bed. And just the thought of taking control of one's life makes any chronically ill patient feel better. The results effectively give the CFS patient more control over her symptoms. When this occurs, the sufferer does better over time.[4] Being in control seems to be important in relieving MS fatigue, so working toward that control with a coach can help the fatigue experienced in MS too. Besides making you feel better by providing you with some control over your illness and by helping you to become more active, the treatment also is effective for depression and for the feeling of demoralization[5]— problems that only worsen CFS symptoms.

It is obvious that factors related to you as a person have an impact on the symptoms you feel and on the illness itself. While these issues are relatively minimal after a brief illness, they probably become pro- gressively more important in an illness of long duration. I feel so strongly about the demonstrated value of this type of intervention that I prescribe it for patients with chronic illness of any sort.

10 ❮ Tips for the Patient

The purpose of the last few chapters has been to help you help yourself cope with stress and its product, fatigue. For those of you whose fatigue is due to stress, using these techniques will solve your problem of fatigue. Unfortunately, others of you will see some improvement from these approaches but will continue to suffer greatly. If you number yourself in these legions, this chapter is for you.

Tip 1: Find a good doctor. In Chapter 5, I laid out the reasons why you may have a problem in achieving this goal. Frequently, you may encounter a doctor characterized by the 3 Bs—brash, boorish, and bullying. It is easy to understand why you might abandon the standard medical approach when you find yourself in the office of this kind of physician—over and over again. Nonetheless, for two major reasons you should stay with a classic medical doctor—someone with the initials M.D. or D.O. (Doctor of Osteopathy) after his or her name. The first is that part of the curriculum of medical school involves learning about the science of medicine. The doctor is required to demand proof, not just opinion. The advantage is that the doctor is less likely to be fooled by statements that such and such a treatment works to "cure" CFS than is a practitioner who has not learned the scientific method. There is nothing wrong with having a skeptical doctor. That kind of person will demand proof and help you understand that believing that something works is not the same as proving it. The second reason is that the classic medical doctor will know about all the new drugs. Say a new medicine is released for insomnia. The doctor will be the only person able to prescribe it for you—not the chiropractor or the homeopath.

The way to find the right doctor for you is to abandon the passive approach. As we approach the year 2000, the physician and the patient are partners. The old parent-child relationship between doctor and patient is disappearing. Obviously, there are still many doctors who want to tell you what to do and expect you to listen without comment. But at least as many doctors are willing to include you in developing an approach to your illness. Today medicine is acknowledged to be big business. We see advertisements extolling such and such a hospital. Medical practices are struggling to arrive at ways to attract more patients. Finding a doctor is a buyer's market. If a doctor is not right for you, that doctor loses you as a patient and as a potential source of income. So when you ask questions, you should expect to get answers. Obviously, you must realize that the doctor only has so much time for you during any one appointment, but some of that time should be devoted to answering your questions.

Since you or your insurance company is paying, you are entitled to a doctor who listens to you and takes your complaints seriously. So if your HMO assigns you to a doctor who has the 3 Bs, tell the case manager or the HMO director that that doctor is not for you. Say that you want a physician who will listen to you and help you with your condition. Finding the doctor with the 3 Cs—caring, communicative, and creative—sometimes takes repeated trial and effort. Or you may hear about such a doctor from an acquaintance who also suffers from chronic fatigue. Good news travels fast. The doctor with the 3 Cs will take your hand and march through time with you. The reason why it is important to have a caring and communicative doctor is self-evident. A creative doctor will do whatever she or he believes is necessary to help you cope with your illness. Being creative means that physician will not be locked into using the prescription pad but will use other medical modalities as well. I often prescribe chiropracty or acupuncture for joint and muscle pain. Then why not skip the middleman and go straight to the chiropractor? Because for some types of pain, that is not a reasonable approach and because I am in touch with the medical advances in understanding and treating CFS. A doctor doesn't have to be any kind of genius to keep up to date; all that is needed is commitment. You deserve a doctor like that.

Tip 2: Be wary of the miracle cure or curer. Over the years, patients have asked my opinion about some medicine that they have heard works miracles in CFS. Several years ago, taking strong antifungal medicines in the belief that CFS was some sort of yeast infestation was not uncommon. Fortunately, that fad has passed, because there is absolutely no evidence that CFS patients have any such infestation. Then there was a great deal of interest in coenzyme Q, which at least is not dangerous (except to your pocketbook). Now patients are asking me about blue-green algae.

The basis for all these stories is that a CFS patient has taken one of these products and has gotten better. The tale spreads like brushfire through the CFS community and everyone wants to try the product. Obviously, if everyone really did get better and CFS disappeared, or if the treatment produced greatly diminished symptoms, trying such products would make a lot of sense. Because CFS is a syndrome of more than one cause, this miraculous result is rarely seen. And no one is willing to do the hard work to prove that such a treatment is effective. A lot of patients try the drug, vitamin, or nutritional aid until something better comes along. Sometimes patients want to try the preparation even if no benefit has been shown in scientific testing.

That is certainly the case for intravenous gamma globulin. If CFS patients had to pay for this medicine themselves (about $5,000 a dose), only a few would ever take it. But since insurance covers the treatment, many patients want to try it. Perhaps my own personal practice is composed of the sickest, most treatment-resistant patients imaginable, but I have not seen one patient definitively improve on this treatment. And I am not alone. A recent paper from Australia could demonstrate no improvement for a group of CFS patients given gamma globulin compared to others given infusions without the immune active material.[1]

How about those nutritional supplements available at health food stores? Just because there is little evidence that these products help in CFS does not mean that not one of them does work. Some certainly could help the CFS sufferer. My rule of thumb is that if the product is not harmful and is not exorbitantly expensive, a six-week trial is reasonable. If at the end of six weeks, you are undecided whether you are any better, you probably are not and you should stop taking the product. It is surprising how rarely this route is followed. Many new patients consulting me for the first time are ingesting more than a dozen food supplements or vitamins. They are very expensive and don't appear to be helpful. The first thing I do is tell the patient to discontinue them, if only to stop needless expenditures.

Some CFS practitioners arrive at nonstandard treatments (such as prescribing antifungals) because they believe they know the cause of CFS. Often the practitioners build their ideas of "cause" from data in the medical literature. A popular focus is the brain—particularly hypothalamo-pituitary function. The illogical leap often made is based on the practitioners' lack of appreciation for the difference between correlation and causation. Just because pituitary abnormalities exist in CFS does not mean that CFS is caused by those abnormalities. A different causative factor could produce CFS and also produce pituitary abnormalities. So replacing the endocrine "abnormality" may do nothing for the patient, and in fact may unbalance the hormonal system.

Other practitioners simply are believers in an unproven idea. One example has to do with vitamins. The idea is that if a tiny amount of vitamins helps some conditions, then a massive amount might help other conditions. The logic here is even weaker than in the treatment of CFS patients with hormones. Furthermore, the problem of side effects mounts as the dose of vitamins escalates.

An additional problem in deciding whether any specific treatment helps or not is the interest and belief of both the practitioner and the patient in the treatment's effectiveness. If the practitioner is a strong adherent of a certain treatment and the patient is desperate for improvement, the chances are that their mutual belief will have a positive therapeutic effect. This is called the placebo effect and it is a powerful therapeutic modality, no matter what the illness. The results from the trial of intravenous immunoglobulin have importance because the researchers compared the effect of the treatment to a placebo and found no differences. This is called a placebo-controlled trial. Practitioners rarely have the time or the devotion to perform carefully controlled, clinical trials of any particular treatment, so relatively ineffective treatments continue to be prescribed for long periods of time. This can be a financial trap for the patient.

Obviously, if there were one or several drug treatments that improved CFS, every practitioner would be using them. My advice to you as a patient is to resist the pat explanation. Or take it to your family doctor and ask for an opinion. Another option is to call Dr. John Renner's consumer health information hot line (816-228-4595). Renner has spent most of the last two decades separating fact from fiction in terms of treatments for illnesses including CFS. My personal advice to patients taking potentially dangerous drugs for ambiguous indications is usually negative; I suggest that the risk outweighs the tiny chance of benefit.

I do think that the doctor who tries a nonstandard or unorthodox treatment is often trying to be creative, and it is possible that some formula will work. Here my rule is the same as for food additives and vitamins: it is all right to try it if the medicine is not dangerous or extremely costly; but if you do try it, stop in six weeks if you are not sure you have gotten any benefit.

Tip 3: Get a coach. I believe anyone with chronic illness needs help in developing coping strategies. There is nothing like talking to an objective, thoughtful person about your problems. That person will have new ideas for you to try. Again, if this approach does not seem to be helping you and several months have gone by, it is time to stop.

Tip 4: Improve your support network. Some patients are luckier than others in that they have a truly understanding family and a set of friends to whom they can turn when they feel dreadful. In contrast, some patients are all alone; their family members think they are lazy, and they have only a limited group of friends. The amount of support that you have influences your ability to cope. In a comparison of one patient to another, the one who has an active support system suffers less than the one who does not.[2]

You are saying to me: "This is the way it is. How can I improve my support system?" There are a number of possibilities. The Internet (alias the Net) provides the simplest solution. It does not matter how disabled you are. If you have a computer and an account with Microsoft, America Online, or some other Internet provider—probably even your telephone company—you are hooked in. You can subscribe (at no cost) to a CFS bulletin board or discussion group. To become part of the CFS newsgroup, you subscribe by e-mailing to <cfs-l@maelstrom.stjohns.edu> the following message: SUB CFS-L yourfirstname yourlastname. The owner of the list then adds your name, and you will see daily postings from other members of the list. Most people subscribe, read the entries to the bulletin board for a while to become familiar with the concept, and then jump in themselves. In one year's time I have seen the CFS bulletin board grow from a hundred postings a month to more than a thousand. People, usually patients, write about whatever they want. Sometimes they ask advice about treatments or they discuss weird symptoms. It doesn't matter. You are hooked into a community that cares about you.

The same thing can happen with a local support group. I believe these are advantageous if they exist to share information. I'm not so sure of their value when they exist for patients to share symptoms. Many patients have told me that the process turned them off. Maybe because it is a lot harder to type than to talk, the postings on the Net are usually short. Even when symptoms are discussed, they seem easier to listen to (or ignore) than when patients relate their symptoms in an actual group. Probably the best groups are the few in which a professional afflicted with the illness acts as coach; then the group gets the benefit of the coach at no cost.

National support and/or information groups are another option. Of all those available, only one prides itself on providing you, the consumer, with scientifically accurate information. That is the National CFS and FM Association, P.O. Box 18426, Kansas City, MO 64133. Writing to the association will get you on a mailing list for its newsletter, but to continue receiving the newsletter you will be asked to join; the cost is $25 per year, tax free.

Another option is a national advocacy group called the Chronic Fatigue and Immune Dysfunction Syndrome (CFIDS) Association of America, P.O. Box 220398, Charlotte, NC 28222-0398; (800) 442-3437. The annual $35 membership fee brings the organization's quarterly magazine. The association provides information on the location of support groups, and it is active politically in trying to get increased federal support for CFS research.

Another powerful source of support requires you to turn to the computer again. In order to access these groups, you need to be part of the World Wide Web. Included in the packet from your Internet provider is a program that will get you onto the Web. Then Web or Net browsers will prompt you to specify certain addresses. When you type them in, you get a number of choices about the item (in this case CFS) in which you are interested.

I can suggest two Web sites for people interested in CFS. I use the Web browser called Netscape, and when its logo comes up on my computer, I see a window that says "Location." Type in the following Web site exactly as follows:

http://www2.infoseek.com/Titles?qt=cfs (then hit carriage return)

This entry calls a Web searcher known as Infoseek into your computer and commands the searcher to go out on the Web and identify any address with "cfs" in it. The last time I did so, Infoseek came up with over seven hundred different addresses, including a very short description of each in the order it deemed most relevant. You are given these ten at a time so that you will not be overwhelmed.

It is possible that your Web provider does not give you access to Infoseek. Another and perhaps an easier way to get started is to let Marc Fluks guide you. Dr. Fluks is a CFS patient at a university in Holland. He has set up a "beginner's guide," which is simply a starting point with subjects on which you can mouse-click to go where you are interested. Among the data easily accessible this way are answers to frequently asked questions (FAQ) about CFS. To get there, type the following Web address:

http://www.dds.nl/~me-net/meweb/begin.html

These two methods are simply different ways of accessing the same information. Both Web addresses will give you the option of finding other self-help and/or bulletin boards beyond the few I have provided in this tip.

If you want the same capability for the illness of Gulf War veterans, type the following:

http://www.dtic.dla.mil/gulflink

Keep in mind that going out on the Net is like going shopping. Buyer beware! What you see is uncensored information. Some of it is based on medical fact; some of it is pure speculation and opinion.

A totally different strategy for improving your support system is to go to church. Obviously, this is not the route if you have no belief in religion or interest in the church. But if you are not absolute in your disbelief, give it a try. Make an appointment with the priest, minister, or rabbi and tell that person a little about yourself and your illness. Don't be surprised when the pastor takes on the role of coach; that kind of training is a critical part of today's pastoral education. One benefit of going to church is the possibility of finding a coach whom you like. Most churches have a place in the service where prayers for the sick are offered. Be sure the pastor includes you in those prayers. It helps to know that people care enough to pray for you. Churches or synagogues are composed of groups of people organized to offer support to one another. Avail yourself of this remarkable service. You will probably feel better for it.

Tip 5: Have a positive attitude. I can just hear you muttering, "That's easy for you to say." Attitude is a lot like social support. If you have a positive attitude, you cope better and your symptoms bother you less than if you have a negative attitude. Some people are born with a positive attitude; others are born with a negative one. In looking at yourself, do you see someone who always sees the glass as half empty, not half full? That is the sign of a negative attitude. How, you are asking, can you change something as basic as that? If those negative attitudes come from the automatic negative thinking discussed in Chapter 9, they can be changed. If you are negative, a coach may turn you around and make you a lot more positive.

Being confronted with illness, disability, and sometimes unsympathetic family could make the most positive person negative. It is normal for such problems to get you down—for you to become de-moralized. Be aware that being demoralized is not the same as being depressed, although demoralization can be a component of depression. In any case, demoralization will certainly impact negatively on your quality of life.

You need to try to cope with this negativism. Being able to discuss it with a friend or a loving family member is one way. Another is attempting to switch from negative thinking to positive thinking. To do this, try to identify one positive happening during your day. Perhaps it is the moment when your head stops throbbing or when a friend comes over to visit. Review your day and find that moment and focus on it. At first it may be hard to find the rewarding moment in the day, but with practice it will be easier. And you may find other positive moments.

For some people, being negative and down in the dumps is an unfortunate habit. Compare yesterday to today. Perhaps nothing good happened to you yesterday, but today you can find something, albeit small, that is positive. That represents improvement and a change in your habit. Some of you may be able to extend this to your illness. If you felt slightly better, even for only a brief time, you can tell yourself at the end of the day, "Today was better than yesterday." By focusing on the positive, you will be able to find something beneficial in the day several times a week. If you get in the habit of accentuating the positive, the negative will diminish. You will feel better.

Tip 6: Laugh. When a patient comes into my office, she usually does not know what to expect. I tell her two things. One is that I am sure I can help her—if only a little. And the second is that she cannot leave my office until she has laughed. Many patients are shocked to hear this, but by the end of our hour and a half together, they will have laughed. Why do I insist on this?

To begin with, the patient gets comfortable with me. It becomes clear to her that I will not be stuffy or paternalistic, and that I will want her to be part of a two-person team aimed at helping with her illness. Even more important, it makes the point that laughter has to be part of the treatment regimen. It provides a way to escape the illness. No one can focus on how awful they feel if they watch one of the ancient but riotously funny Marx Brothers movies. If the Marx Brothers don't do it, perhaps Roseanne will. The point is that laughing is positive, whereas weeping is negative. Putting more ticks on the positive side makes coping easier and reduces symptoms.

Tip 7: If you are disabled, be persistent with the authorities. CFS patients diagnosed by the 1988 case definition are often unable to live normal lives. In fact, over half the patients in our research pool are unable to work. For patients in white-collar jobs, the reasons often relate to fatigue and cognitive difficulties. For patients doing more physically demanding jobs, the reasons often relate again to fatigue, and to symptom flareups following exertion. The question is, how do you deal with disability?

When patients come to me and lay out the reasons why they cannot work, I grimace to myself because the prognosis for recovery is always better when the patient can remain in the workplace—if only on a part-time basis. But disability is often a part of severe fatiguing illness. Some of the tips I have already listed should help you deal psychologically with this life change. But if your company lets you go, or if you are too sick to return to work, you need to start the disability remuneration process.

Obtaining disability benefits for an illness that has no specific laboratory abnormality is often a frustrating journey, but at least in the United States, if there is adequate evidence that you can no longer report to work regularly, the journey will eventually end. The relationship with your physician is critical. If your doctor does not recognize that you are ill, his letter to your insurance company, to your employer, or to the Social Security Administration will reflect that. If the doctor does appreciate your illness, often a mountain of paper has to be built to help you on your journey. Letters are required stating that you are disabled and listing the reasons for the disability. The disability agency asks the doctor's opinion about your performance of physical tasks like bending, crawling, and carrying. Preparing these letters is not an easy task for a busy doctor, and the requesting agencies pay the doctor very little for the time it takes to draft them. So, if you are unable to work, you will have to discuss the process of obtaining benefits with your doctor. If he is unwilling to support you, it is time once more to seek another doctor. In my experience, when a patient is too sick to work and has a caring doctor, disability status from an insurance company or from the government eventually is forthcoming.

11 (The Medical Treatment of Psychological Causes of Fatigue

If you feel fine one day and wake up the next in an incredibly fatigued state that does not go away in a few days, surely you will go to your doctor for help. If, however, she finds no medical cause for your illness, you may be left to your own devices. At this point, additional medical consultation is probably not the road to take. Assuming that your fatigue is caused by stress or anxiety, going to medically oriented care givers with the complaint of fatigue at that time is likely not to be productive in that the course they will choose will probably be the one I have laid out in prior chapters. But if you have begun a stress-management program and are doing some aerobic exercise and have shown no improvement, then it is time to make an appointment with your doctor.

Chapters 7, 8, and 9 have dealt with the most common cause of fatigue—stress. The feelings produced by stress are very much the same as in the psychiatric ailment known as anxiety. The difference is that we usually know what it is that produces the feelings of stress, whereas with anxiety the feelings seem to come out of the blue. All the same, anxiety has the same effect as stress: it produces fatigue. Anxiety responds to the same treatments as stress. Stress is not a lifelong phenomenon, but anxiety can be. Therefore, while many people with stress and anxiety will find help in the program laid out in previous chapters, some will not. These are the people who will have to return to the doctor for medical treatment. In the past, doctors prescribed tranquilizers for stress or anxiety—the Valium-type drugs whose pharmaceutical family name is the benzodiazepines. However, many of these drugs may lose their efficacy in relieving anxiety if given for prolonged periods of time, can produce fatigue on their own, and also introduce the risk of dependence. These drugs can be hard to stop because the body gets used to your taking them. For these reasons, doctors usually prescribe benzodiazepines if the anxiety is expected to be short lived. If I suspect underlying anxiety is producing fatigue, I eschew these drugs for a drug called Buspar. This tranquilizer is not in the same class of drugs as Valium. Patients taking it can quickly taper off without uncomfortable side effects.

Because of the problems related to the Valium-type drugs, I rarely begin with them when I am treating patients whose fatigue does not appear to be due to anxiety. Yet, I have had patients consult with me who were taking these medicines as prescribed by their previous doctor. Surprisingly, some patients say these medicines energize them rather than fatigue them. So it is possible that this class of drugs does have a role in the treatment of chronic fatigue. But when a drug has an opposite action from its usual one, I become concerned. How will we ever figure out what this drug is doing? However, if a patient feels better and understands the issues involved in taking these drugs for a long time, I will prescribe them until the patient believes they are no longer working.

The other major psychological cause of fatigue is depression. Depression and anxiety would seem to be worlds apart: the anxious person is nervous and agitated, while the depressed person is withdrawn, sad, and quiet. But the two psychiatric conditions share one element:

many of the medicines that relieve symptoms of one disorder relieve symptoms of the other disorder too.

This is certainly true for the antidepressant medications. No one antidepressant works any better than the next, except that the newer ones are far freer from side effects than the older versions. Recent work has demonstrated that some of the older antidepressants such as Tofranil reduce symptoms of anxiety also.[1] While newer-generation antidepressants such as Prozac were originally thought to have an opposite effect, researchers now feel that these drugs too are able to relieve the symptoms of anxiety.

Until recently, my own treatment plan was to try a low or normal dose of one of the new-generation antidepressants on anyone with unexplained chronic fatigue, as a "therapeutic trial" for masked depression. Several careful studies, however, suggest that these drugs relieve neither chronic fatigue nor fibromyalgia.[2] Of the many hundreds of patients I have seen with chronic fatigue syndrome and/or fibromyalgia, I can remember only one who had no suggestion of depression and who was greatly helped by treatment with Prozac, the first of these new-generation antidepressants that was marketed. So I have changed my practice accordingly: I no longer prescribe these medicines if I find no evidence of significant depression. Remember, not everyone with chronic illness has depression.

What about when depression is obvious? The available information is ambiguous. In the study on CFS, Prozac did not improve coexisting depression; but in the study on fibromyalgia, it did.[3] Although our group has been in the forefront of those arguing that the depression seen in fatiguing illness is different from that seen in major depressive disorder, I still believe that CFS or fibromyalgia depression can be treated. So I will try this class of medicines. Since I do not have placebo controls, I can never be sure of the results. Quite often, though, my patients tell me that their fatigue remains the same, but that their outlook toward the illness has improved. To me, that response is a valid reason for trying these drugs.

I have been talking about Prozac, the prototype of this class of drugs. A number of similar drugs have recently entered the market. Their major advantage is that they remain in the body for a far shorter time than Prozac. It takes about a month for all traces of Prozac to disappear, which is a problem for patients who develop allergies or adverse reactions to the drug. Still, it is important to understand that Prozac and similar drugs are not miracle workers. No one antidepressant is more effective than another. The principal difference is that the new drugs are cleaner; they relieve depression with fewer side effects. And some of the side effects that remain can be helpful. For instance, Prozac tends to be activating, which helps some patients with severe fatigue. However, it can be too activating and make patients nervous. Again, the only difference among the antidepressants on the market is the side effects they cause. In terms of treating depression, one is the equivalent of the other.

Your physician will go over the side effects with you during a consultation. A rash is probably the worst, but nausea, anxiety, sexual dysfunction, and fatigue itself may also occur. Side effects of the new antidepressants occur on an individual basis, but they are not the rule. I attempt to reduce the chances for side effects by starting with half of the recommended dose. Not starting at the full dose given to seriously depressed people seems reasonable to me. After all, if you have had your problem for more than six months, it does not make sense to try to get rid of it in a week or two. Starting low and going slow is the more sensible course of action. When, despite this strategy, side effects emerge, I simply change drugs. The proliferation of these new-generation antidepressants makes it possible to tailor treatment to the individual patient.

For some of you, treatment of depression will end your fatiguing

illness. But for those of you with chronic fatigue syndrome, it probably will not. Prior to moving on to treatments for CFS, let me make
the very important point that depression acts to make any physical
illness worse. It does not matter whether it is Alzheimer's disease,
heart failure, or terminal cirrhosis; when depression is present, you
will feel worse and fare worse. For some people—fortunately not all—
physical illness brings depression. That does not mean your illness is
"all in your head." It simply means that the depression must be treated
in order to help you cope better and to begin reducing the intensity of
your physical discomfort. Your physician and your coach can help
you achieve this goal.

12 (The Medical Treatment of Chronic Fatiguing Illnesses

Chronic illness carries its own baggage. When you are well one minute and sick the next and when the sickness does not go away, you change. Chronic fatiguing illnesses such as CFS are not like AIDS, which is lethal; CFS is disabling—you change overnight from a well person to a sick person. Experiencing that change brings other changes. You become more dependent on those around you, which is difficult to accept if you have never had to do this before. You may deny that you have a chronic illness and push yourself when you should rest. All these changes can be magnified by two other factors: how you feel physically and mentally, and how others feel about you.

Let me explain. The first is easy. The sicker you are, the harder it is to escape the obvious fact that your life has changed. Similarly, if your illness has made you depressed, it is hard to cope in a positive way. You do things that are self-defeating—for example, you cut yourself off from friends whose help you may need. The second element that causes problems for patients with chronic fatiguing illness is rejection. A time may come when some member or members of your family accuse you of being lazy or of shirking your normal duties. They will tell you that enough is enough and it is time to go back to work. Such rejection makes everything worse and increases your insecurity, because you are not sure yourself just what your problem is. The same sequence may happen with your doctor. You make an appointment and your physician either tells you there is really nothing wrong with you, that you should see a psychiatrist with the idea that you have an emotional problem, or that there simply is nothing that can be done for you. Either way, this constitutes another rejection and leaves you in charge of yourself and coping with your illness—alone. Again, the results of rejection by your doctor magnify your symptoms, make any depression worse, and increase your problems in coping with chronic illness. Obviously, these are all reasons for a coach; but at this point you probably need a doctor, too.

The Right Doctor
Finding a doctor who listens to you and does not tell you that there is nothing wrong or that nothing can be done for you is the first step in feeling better. A professional who will listen to you and respond to you positively will make you feel better. Dealing with rejection—from family or physician—takes energy. Acceptance produces positive feelings and makes you feel better immediately.

The second step has to do with diagnosis. Early versions of the case definition of CFS provided the physician the information needed to make the diagnosis. But what about the patient with fatiguing illness who did not meet the criteria? She and her physician were left to figure out a diagnosis. The 1994 publication of an international consensus group's criteria for dealing with fatiguing illness helped to remedy this problem.[1] The physician now has a plan for how to deal with fatiguing illness. You will be diagnosed and will no longer have the terrible feeling of not knowing what your problem is. It is amazing how giving something a name—even a vague name like CFS—makes a patient feel better.

One Approach to Treatment

The third step has to do with treatment and is at the heart of this chapter. Because there is no specific treatment for chronic fatigue syndrome, physicians each develop their own ways of improving the health and quality of life of the CFS patient. Before I tell you how I treat CFS, you should understand my perspective. I am a professor at a medical school. In that role, I teach students what I consider to be the proper way to practice medicine. To put it concisely, I believe the doctor's job is to do anything within the realm of medical knowledge to help his or her patient. If there is no strong logic or reason for any specific treatment, or at least rudimentary evidence that some newly conceived treatment works, I will not use it. So no intravenous vitamin drips, no antifungals, no pituitary hormones, no "immune stimulants." I am not being negative: I am simply unwilling to teach my students that using flimsy logic to develop an uncontrolled treatment plan is valid (or even adequate) medicine. Because of this attitude, I am unwilling to suggest such a treatment plan to persons who are suffering—despite their need and hope for a therapeutic solution. My patients seem to appreciate my efforts to be logical and honest with them, so I continue doing things my way.

In contrast to my approach, some physicians will follow any logic, no matter how tenuous, to develop a treatment and will continue to treat unless or until the treatment demonstrably makes the patient worse. I worry that this approach carries with it high costs for the patient, both financially and psychologically, should the treatment not produce its promised benefits. Although not always the case, university-based physicians tend to use treatment rules similar to the ones I will now lay out.

Since there is no specific remedy for CFS, my treatment focuses on relieving the symptoms of the illness. When I ask patients with chronic fatiguing illness to tell me which symptom they would most like to lose, I usually get one of two complex answers: either the

fatigue, the sick feeling that comes with it, and the difficulty in concentrating, thinking, and performing on the job *or* relief from pain in
head, muscles, or joints.

Blood Tests

I ask patients this question at the end of my first meeting with them to
help me better understand their problem. At that first visit I carefully
review their previous medical evaluation and ask for additional blood
testing if all the tests that I think are required to rule out other medical
causes of fatigue have not been done. In addition to the standard
blood count, urinalysis, thyroid testing, and body chemistries, I look
for signs of chronic mild irritation or inflammation of body tissues
with tests called the sed (sedimentation) rate and a test of muscle
chemistry called creatine phosphokinase, abbreviated as CPK. Very
high sed rates point to a lupus-like illness; high CPKs point to muscle
disease. If the patient has one of these diagnoses, she does not have
CFS.

Because Lyme disease is so prevalent in my region, I repeat that
test. Should the laboratory find a positive result, I draw another tube
of blood and mail it to the immunology laboratory at the State University of New York's medical school at Stony Brook. Lyme is a problem on which they concentrate at that center; if your doctor thinks it
is indicated, she or he can arrange to send a specimen of your blood
there (516-444-3824). Finally, I do screening tests for HIV disease,
lupus, and rheumatoid arthritis.

I often do one other test to determine if the levels of magnesium
are normal in the blood cells. An English group reported that levels of
this element can be low in chronic fatiguing illnesses, and that patients can feel better when they are given magnesium shots to restore
their levels to normal.[2] I must tell you immediately that the report of
low red-blood-cell magnesium in patients with CFS has not been
replicated and other groups have not had the same success in treating

with magnesium shots. In my own experience it rarely is successful, but it is a simple treatment whose major side effect is that the shots hurt! So when I find patients whose red-blood-cell magnesium is low, I recommend a trial of weekly magnesium injections for a six-week period. When patients have red cell magnesium toward the bottom of the normal range, I ask them to take oral magnesium glycinate for six weeks with the goals of reducing symptoms and raising levels to the high range of normal. Why not oral magnesium for everyone? Because it is very poorly absorbed and often produces diarrhea.

Although the English group claimed that giving these shots helped all their patients, that was obviously not my experience. But perhaps for the occasional patient, the magnesium will work. I use the same line of thought relative to primrose oil and fish oil. One report in the medical literature claims that taking these substances on a daily basis relieves severe fatiguing illness.[3] Other groups have done careful testing to try to confirm the beneficial effect of these oils but have been unsuccessful. To a scientist, that means that the use of these oils as a treatment for fatiguing illness is at best questionable. But in my opinion, the doctor's responsibility to the patient exceeds the necessity to be totally scientific. After all, the oils could help a small percentage of patients with chronic fatiguing illness. So I recommend that the patient try these oils for a six-week period. The only real side effect I have found is nausea or upset stomach from the fish oil. For thirty or forty dollars, a trial of these oils seems reasonable. Six weeks is my cut-off point for any of these unvalidated treatments. If at the end of that time the patient is quite sure that she has improved, we continue treatment. If not, we stop.

By the time the patient comes for a follow-up visit, I have the results of the laboratory tests and, when appropriate, I can make the diagnosis of CFS or some other ailment. What I do next is determine whether the oils or the magnesium has helped. If so, I offer no further treatment. However, I have yet to see either of these medicines "cure" someone with chronic fatiguing illness. My best result has been some improvement. Of course, the patients I see tend to be very ill and often disabled. Perhaps less seriously affected patients with fatiguing illness would do better on one of these treatments.

If a patient has no medical explanation for severe and chronic fatigue, I often draw additional blood at this time to test it for a hormone called DHEA and for one of its metabolites, DHEA-S. A hormone made in the adrenal gland, DHEA is used frequently in Europe as a tonic to treat fatigue. It is attracting a lot of attention because it may slow some of the usual consequences of aging.[4] Although a group at Temple University has noted that levels of this hormone can be elevated in CFS, I have never found high levels in any of the CFS patients I have tested. Instead, I have found an occasional CFS patient whose DHEA or DHEA-S level is below normal. When I prescribe 25 to 50 milligrams of DHEA to such patients, a few have reported significant and long-lasting relief. This natural substance is now available in health food stores but, again, there are questions about purity and dosage. Your doctor can get you capsules of pharmaceutical-grade hormone by calling one of the following pharmacies: 800-888-9358 or 800-792-6670. Although the number of patients who have low levels of this hormone is small, and the number of patients who respond to treatment is even smaller, I still check all patients' levels because the side effects of this drug are rare. When they do occur, they appear as acne or a tendency for increased body hair growth; very rarely, they can affect the liver. With DHEA too, I follow the six-week rule.

Neurogenic Postural Hypotension
As I was writing this book, a new idea arose about the cause of CFS. A group at Johns Hopkins Medical School noted that, in contrast to healthy people, many CFS patients felt as if they were going to faint when they were tilted into an upright position.[5] Lightheadedness or

dizziness is common in CFS, and patients often report that their fatigue gets worse if they have to remain on their feet for more than a few minutes.

The tendency to faint is associated with a drop in blood pressure, which is called hypotension. It is normal for blood pressure to fall somewhat when you stand up. Blood briefly pools in the legs and so less is available in the rest of the body. The normal response to this brief drop is the triggering of a reflex to maintain blood pressure in the rest of the body. If the reflex does not achieve this end, blood flow to the brain diminishes. If blood flow is sufficiently low, the patient loses consciousness; this is fainting.[6]

To probe this normal physiological reaction to postural challenge, the Hopkins researchers used a two-part protocol—tilt alone, then tilt in the presence of an intravenously infused drug that dilates the blood vessels and thus additionally stresses the system. Because of their finding that many CFS patients felt substantially less fatigued after treatment for this "neurogenic hypotension," the Hopkins group concluded that at least some CFS patients have severe fatigue due to an abnormality in this reflex.

The usual pattern for people who have difficulties with this reflex is a rapid drop in blood pressure with tilting. The Hopkins group found a different pattern, one in which the patient in head-up tilt did just fine until many minutes had passed. This sort of abnormality is seen most often in younger people and those whose resting blood pressure tends to be on the low side. Another indicator is a high heart rate, especially in the standing posture. The successful results of treating the posturally related hypotension quickly made national news. Since doctors could do nothing to strengthen the reflex, their tactic was to increase the amount of fluid in the patients' blood vessels to reduce the possibility of blood pooling in the limbs during postural challenge.

This work focused my attention on two things: patient complaints of dizziness, especially when related to changes in posture, and either low blood pressure or high heart rate at rest. These can be indicators of posturally related hypotension. In a few cases I have sent patients for tilt testing and they have had abnormal results. However, there are problems with tilt testing: first, it is often positive in healthy people, especially when intravenous drugs are given to increase the chance of producing fainting,[7] and, second, CFS patients are frequently on medicines like Elavil, which themselves can produce postural hypotension and thus increase the chance of abnormal tilt testing. At our center the experience with tilt testing is that it is positive as often in sedentary healthy people as it is in CFS patients. To me this means the test is at best insensitive. What is the patient (and the doctor) to do until these complications are sorted out?

Since the only known marker for this neurally mediated hypotension is intolerance to tilt testing, my indications for a therapeutic trial are use of tilt testing in conjunction with symptoms of dizziness and/or increased fatigue when standing. My initial treatment utilizes a conservative approach, focused on the symptom of dizziness. If it follows postural change or if the resting blood pressure is low, I tell the patient to increase salt intake. Why salt? Because salt carries water with it and therefore puts more fluid in the blood vessels. More blood is then available to keep the brain working while the patient is in the upright posture. How to increase salt intake? By eating everything that you might otherwise *not* eat—for instance, pickles, pretzels, soup made from bouillon cubes, and potato chips. When increased salt intake is difficult to achieve via diet, salt tablets are a reasonable alternative. Since salt ingestion can influence resting blood pressure and kidney function, your physician should be involved when you try this protocol.

Another simple way to help yourself is to wear support stockings. They compress the blood vessels in the legs, thereby reducing the likelihood of blood pooling in the legs when you are standing.

My last suggestion is that patients prop up the head of their bed by putting a brick under each of the two legs; this is the strategy I suggested in Chapter 6 to reduce acid reflux into the esophagus. Sleeping with a slight head-up tilt makes assuming the upright posture less of a stress on the cardiovascular system. If these conservative treatments help, fine. But what if the symptoms continue and the tilt test is positive?

Here a trial of medicine is indicated. Reports in the medical literature indicate that drugs of surprisingly different modes of action all work in this condition, a fact that raises a lot of questions. For example, a number of short notes in the literature indicate that the new "low side effect" antidepressants such as Prozac can be effective. Do they treat the posturally related hypotension, or is this postural problem an accompaniment to some forms of depression? That information does not exist. Since a trial of such a drug might also treat any underlying depression, one Prozac a day for the CFS patient with a positive tilt test seems reasonable. As with other trials, I use my six-week rule. If the medicine is not effective and the patient continues to have major posturally related symptoms, I turn to other therapeutic alternatives.

The first, Fluorinef, makes the body retain salt and water and actually expands the amount of blood in the vasculature. With more blood in the vessels, more blood is available to the brain even if pooling in the legs takes place. Since it is the relative absence of blood in the brain that causes fainting, the treatment protects the brain and the posturally related symptoms lessen. Unfortunately, this medicine has many side effects (swelling, worse fatigue, nausea, headaches, more dizziness, depression) and is often very difficult to take. This is especially a problem in that as many as three pills per day (0.1 milligram each) may be required for improvement. Although I am willing to try this drug, it usually presents so many problems that it is rare for me to keep patients on it for months or even weeks.

Because side effects are such a problem for patients using this powerful drug in CFS—even at the very low starting dose of a quarter-tablet of the 0.1 milligram pill—I have turned to trials of licorice extract. Licorice has many of the same effects as Fluorinef in producing salt and water retention, but it seems to be much gentler. In using licorice, I am acting as a doctor and not as a scientist, because I do not know how effective the drug is at the dose used. The lack of significant side effects may simply mean that the dosage is too low. But some of my patients insist that they feel better for having taken it. Your physician can get the five-to-one solid extract in 4-ounce bottles by prescription from Scientific Botanicals (206-527-5521), or a local pharmacy can obtain the preparation for your doctor from that supplier.

I start with a quarter of a teaspoon per day, and I have increased the dosage to as much as three times a day. Since one of the actions of both licorice and Fluorinef is also to reduce potassium, I prescribe a potassium supplement for patients while they are on these medicines. Low potassium worsens the side effects of Fluorinef. These preparations function by altering the amounts of sodium and potassium salts in the body, and these salts are the materials on which cellular function depends. Therefore, use of such medications requires close monitoring by your physician.

Another treatment uses a class of drugs called beta-blockers. Usually these are given to reduce blood pressure, an action which would seem contrary to what is desired for our purposes. However, another action of these medicines is to stop the pooling of blood in the legs when a patient is standing. This action then can block the tendency for dizziness or faintness when CFS patients stand up. Again my rule is a six-week trial. If the patient reports real improvement, I will continue treatment; if not, I will stop.

Another treatment with a drug called midodrine, and sold as Pro-Amatine, became available in late 1996. At the time of writing, I have not had occasion to use this drug, but it has been successfully employed in groups of patients with neurogenic postural hypotension.[8] The drug is converted into a biologically active form that directly constricts blood vessels. If too much is given, or if the drug works too effectively, the result would be an elevation of the blood pressure— perhaps to dangerous levels. A potential problem exists if patients taking ProAmatine also take cold or allergy remedies that have drugs such as phenylephrine or pseudephedrine in them. These drugs relieve nasal congestion by constricting the blood vessels, and this action could supplement that of ProAmatine to raise blood pressure even further. It is clear that hand tailoring of these drugs by the doctor is critical. Doing so often permits combinations of drugs at relatively low doses of each, so that side effects are less of a problem.

One other treatment uses a potent new drug called Epogen to increase the amount of blood in the vessels by stimulating the production of blood cells. The approach is logical, but a study of how it works in practice has not yet been done. The drug is generally used to treat low blood counts or anemias. Patients with CFS, by definition, do not have anemias because, as I indicated in Chapter 2, anemia itself can produce chronic fatigue. The utilization of Epogen to increase the blood cell count in people whose blood counts are already on the high side could be dangerous. Yet it is not unreasonable to consider this treatment in patients with neurogenic hypotension, with blood counts on the low end of normal, and who have not benefited from any of the other treatments discussed. Even in cases such as these, the patient and her doctor must do a cost-benefit analysis; the drug is costly, must be administered by injection, and can take as much as several months for an effect to occur.

Until we know more about posturally related hypotension, I do not believe the approach I have described is indicated for patients who do not have major difficulty with the symptoms. For such patients and for patients with postural symptoms who remain sick despite treatment, other treatment is required. I stress to my patients that we are looking for improvement, unfortunately not for cure. My goal in using any particular medicine is to reduce pain and suffering and allow the patient to lead a more normal life. If a medicine makes a patient 5 percent better, that is real improvement and validates its use.

Depression

When my evaluation even suggests the possibility of depression, I begin a low dose of Prozac (half of the normal suggested daily dose of 20 milligrams). You may ask why I am doing this in light of the study showing that Prozac has no effect on concurrent depression in CFS patients or on their CFS symptoms.[9] Basically, I am unwilling to become a therapeutic nihilist based on one study, even though it seems to have been well conceived and executed. Another study has been done on the effects of Prozac in patients with fibromyalgia. Although it is impossible to know the fatigue status of the patients from the information provided, the study did find a reduction in depression scores for the patients who were treated.[10]

The issue is that the presence of depression makes everything worse, and patients with chronic fatigue can cope much better with their illness if they do not have a simultaneous problem with depression. At the time I start Prozac, I discuss with the patient what symptoms might disappear if the drug is working. Reduction in the number of bouts of crying, lessening of the heavy feeling of sadness and demoralization, and more interest in activities unrelated to illness are specific areas I target. If the patient at the next visit says that one or more of these symptoms is less of a problem, I may increase the drug to the normal daily dose to see if further improvement takes place. Because depression is not uncommon in CFS, Prozac is often the first drug I try. But if the patient returns after a six-week trial and tells me that the medicine has not helped, of course I stop it. When side effects interfere with this trial, I turn to one of the other new antidepressants such as Paxil, Effexor, Wellbutrin, Serzone, or Zoloft.

Our center has done two therapeutic trials with drugs called mono-amine oxidase inhibitors (MAOIs), which were among the early drugs available to treat depression. Our first trial used an antidepressant called Nardil, but at one-quarter of the usual antidepressant dose. To minimize the possibility that any therapeutic effect might simply be due to the antidepressant action of the drug, we excluded patients with obvious depression. Most medical practitioners are uncomfortable using MAOIs to treat depression because the drugs are somewhat difficult to use. If a patient taking these drugs ingests aged or processed food, cheese, or wine, a striking and potentially life-threatening eleva-tion in blood pressure can occur. This toxicity is called the cheese effect. Although it was our belief that this problem would not occur at the dose we used, we counseled our volunteer CFS patients to exclude the foods that might trigger this reaction.

Our second trial used a drug called Eldepryl. Unlike Nardil, El-depryl is a MAOI that does not interact dangerously with foods at the dose prescribed. The drug is approved for Parkinson's disease, but evi-dence does exist that the drug also improves cognitive function.[11] We found that both Nardil and Eldepryl helped, but the effect was quite small. We had hoped that the drugs might improve the functional status of our CFS patients and reduce their disability. Although this was not the case, the small improvement was a step toward improved health. With both these medicines a dangerous interaction with anti-depressant medications is possible. And as I will show you, the anti-depressants have roles in CFS other than altering mood, so they have an important place in the symptomatic management of CFS.

Pain and Insomnia
In fact, some antidepressants relieve patients of complaints of pain and sleeplessness. One treatment that works well for both complaints is a very low dose of one of the old-fashioned antidepressants. Why these medicines alleviate pain is unknown, but they do help! If the

antidepressant dose of one of these medicines is 100 to 150 milligrams, I will start with 10 milligrams, increase to 25 milligrams, and on occasion go as high as 50 or 75 milligrams. If a patient also has problems with insomnia, I will prescribe amitriptyline. If the patient has pain but relatively little problem with sleeplessness, I will use amitriptyline's first cousin, desipramine, which is less sedating. A low dose of amitriptyline can relieve headache as well as muscle and joint pain, and also help the patient fall asleep. A recent study looked at the effects of Prozac alone, amitriptyline alone, and both drugs together in nondepressed patients with fibromyalgia.[12] The researchers concluded that either drug alone improved sleep and sense of well-being, and also reduced pain. The best outcome occurred when patients were taking both of these drugs.

Sometimes a patient will tell me that amitriptyline has helped sleep somewhat, but not enough. Or a patient will tell me that the side effects of the old-line antidepressants are just too much. When that is the case and when relaxation methods do not seem to be enough, I will prescribe a trial first with melatonin and then with Ambien. If these treatments still do not produce improvement in sleep, I will stop the melatonin and add to the Ambien half the normal recommended dose of one of the Valium-type drugs. Specifically, I will use temazepam (15 milligrams) or triazolam (0.125 milligram). With one of these supplementing my other treatments, a reasonable night's sleep is usually possible.

The problem with these medicines is the side effects. Some patients have no problems, others complain mightily. The side effect that probably concerns patients most is weight gain. Often the combination of a low dose, careful weight monitoring, and exercise is all that is needed to bypass this problem. When that does not work, I abandon these medicines and use others to treat insomnia and pain separately. A drug called Meridia could change the equation. It is a weakly active antidepressant that causes people to lose weight. At the time of writing it was not fully approved by the Food and Drug Administration, but when available it may prove ideal in reducing weight gain of patients on these sedating antidepressants.

Another side effect for some people is constipation. Again, low doses of the drugs plus a high-fiber diet usually are enough to allow this kind of treatment. Sometimes too these medicines make the heart race and worsen a tendency toward posturally related symptoms. If one particular medicine disagrees with a patient, I often try another in the same family. Others that relieve pain and insomnia include doxepin and trazadone. Another that resembles desipramine in producing less sedation is nortriptyline.

If some relief occurs but more is needed, I will try other drugs. For pain, I will suggest ibuprofen or Advil. These are in the class of non-steroidal anti-inflammatory drugs (NSAIDs). By definition, inflammation must be present for these drugs to work, and there is no evidence for inflammation in the form of swelling or redness in either CFS or fibromyalgia. Pain relief from this class of drugs is highly variable from patient to patient. For some patients, they definitely help, but for the majority they do not greatly relieve the pain of fibromyalgia. It is possible that they may be more helpful in combination with drugs like amitriptyline.[13]

One of the problems is that patients frequently are taking lower doses than I might prescribe. I give patients with substantial pain high doses of this medicine—as much as four Advil four times a day. Again, the problem is side effects. The medicine must be given with meals and even when it is, an upset stomach is not uncommon. Sometimes when ibuprofen is a problem, the doctor can try another medicine in the same family, but the side effects usually cannot be dodged. If a patient's stomach cannot tolerate these medicines, certainly they cannot be used. At high doses a patient must be under a doctor's care, because taking these medicines for long periods can produce kidney problems and gastric irritation with bleeding.

Fatigue and Confusion

The other problem area about which patients complain is difficulty with concentration and attention. My approach is to explain to the patient that in our careful studies of mental function in CFS, patients do almost as well as healthy, normal people. They are sensing problems that indeed exist, but that are not as intense as they seem. Knowing this helps a bit. But we have also learned that a specific problem area for the CFS patient occurs when she is in a situation where many different auditory inputs are occurring at the same time, say at a party or in a busy cafeteria. The CFS patient seems to do worse in this situation than otherwise healthy patients. In fact, the patient has the same degree of difficulty with this task as a patient with mild multiple sclerosis. Thus I counsel the patient to try to limit activities to situations where she can talk and/or work one-on-one.

While these approaches help, they usually do not suffice to alleviate adequately the patient complaint of impaired mental function. Here again, pharmacological intervention sometimes helps. My approach is to try to treat the fatigue and, by so doing, relieve the complaint of mental fogginess. One treatment initially thought to be useful was a medicine called amantidine, used to prevent viral infection. A number of studies suggested it could be used to relieve the fatigue that is so common in patients with multiple sclerosis. A recent definitive study in which a sugar pill was used as a basis for comparison showed that the medicine did in fact reduce MS fatigue.[14] Although the drug has a place in the treatment of MS fatigue, I have not been impressed by its usefulness in CFS.

Other Difficulties

At this point in treatment, I begin to focus on the individual problems bothering the patient. Usually the combination of relaxation and drug treatment relieves headaches, at least enough so that other problems become worse. If headaches remain a problem, I use one of the other headache remedies. The most common are the beta-blockers, which I have mentioned as a possible treatment for postural dizziness. On occasion I try a medicine called Diamox. Diamox does the opposite of Fluorinef: It forces the kidney to lose salt and water. This process causes a decrease in swelling throughout the body, which sometimes relieves headaches.

Migraine Headaches

If the headaches fluctuate from one side of the head to the other, are pounding, and are preceded by visual blurring or odd visual patterns, they are migrainous. These respond extremely well to a new oral medicine called Imitrex. However, the drug is very expensive. Before I prescribe Imitrex, I usually try 4 percent Lidocaine nose drops. Lidocaine works in the same way as the local anesthetic your dentist uses to prevent pain while he or she is operating on your teeth. In the context of migraines, the patient lies with head hanging off the edge of the bed and turned forty-five degrees toward the side of the pain. Positioning the head in this way allows the anesthetic to bathe nerves that go to the internal coverings of the skull, which are extremely pain sensitive. Blocking these nerves can stop headache pain within minutes.

Muscle and Joint Pain

This brings me back to muscle and joint pain. Frequently, treatment with Prozac, amitriptyline, and NSAIDs still leaves the patient with substantial pain. What then? I then turn to two relatively new drugs: Ultram, which is a nonnarcotic pain reliever, and Neurontin, which is marketed primarily as an antiepileptic but also has a role in chronic pain. For the Ultram, I use the usual recommended doses. For the Neurontin, I start with 100 milligrams before bedtime, as the drug can be sedating, then gradually increase to 400 milligrams before bedtime. If the patient experiences some relief but still is suffering, I will experiment with additional doses during the daytime too, if sedation is not too much of a problem. Some doctors prescribe even higher doses.

Our understanding of what produces pain in CFS or FM is changing. Originally, the pain was thought to represent inflammation of muscle and its fibrous connections to bone. Time has not provided evidence to prove this theory, so FM is thought to be a syndrome of hyperpathia or increased pain.[15] One fact complicates this conclusion, and that is the overlap between fibromyalgia and real inflammatory rheumatic diseases such as lupus erythematosis; the diffuse pain and sensitivity to pressure indicative of FM is a frequent occurrence in lupus.[16] How do doctors determine if there is an inflammatory component in the patient with diffuse pain? They look for evidence of redness or swelling in joints, or pain that is specific to the joint and not to the bone adjoining it. Additional evidence for inflammation is laboratory tests outside the normal range for antinuclear antibodies or rheumatoid factor.

When I suspect underlying inflammation, I then turn to two medicines used by doctors who care for patients with diseases of their joints. One class of these medicines is usually used to treat malaria. During World War II, service personnel in the Pacific were given a drug called atabrine to prevent malaria. Three side effects were quickly noted: the medicine, being a dye, turned the skin yellow; it relieved fatigue; and it also relieved any problems with achy joints. Because of this, the antimalarials were tried in joint pain that resulted from rheumatoid arthritis and they were found to work. The reason for their efficacy is unknown, but one possibility is that they reduce the pain.[17]

Atabrine was only partially effective and had the disadvantage of being a skin dye with other toxic side effects, so attention shifted to a medicine called Plaquenil. Again the problem of side effects arose. This medicine can affect vision. Although such an outcome is very rare, the possibility requires any patient taking Plaquenil to see an ophthalmologist regularly. The usual dose in rheumatological disorders is 6 milligrams per kilogram. If more is required, I work closely with a rheumatologist, expert at use of this medicine.

If these drugs work by reducing pain rather than by reducing inflammation, then there is a real role for them in CFS and FM pain. We can only hope that someone will do a placebo-controlled trial very soon.

Steroid Trials

The principal adrenal steroid hormone, hydrocortisone, was noted to be lower than normal in CFS patients.[18] When this hormone is at extremely low levels, the diagnosis of Addison's disease is made. Patients with Addison's disease have a great deal of fatigue and many symptoms comparable to CFS. Because of the possibility that CFS patients could be helped by treating them with low levels of hydrocortisone to normalize their blood levels, Dr. Steven Straus of the National Institutes of Health (NIH) recently completed a double-blind, placebo-controlled study on seventy CFS patients. Although the thirty-five patients receiving hydrocortisone tended to do better than the thirty-five placebo-treated controls, the small difference could have occurred simply by chance. Because the treated patients did show reduced adrenal function at the end of the twelve-week trial, Straus concluded that the minimal advantage of treatment was offset by the risks of even further reduction in adrenal function. Steroid replacement therapy does not appear to be indicated in CFS.

Investigators at the University of Oregon did a placebo-controlled trial of a stronger medicine in this class, called prednisone, in patients with FM. It did not help.[19] Despite this result, I do a short-term trial of this drug in patients whose muscle and joint pains have not been helped by all the other treatment options. Prednisone is an example of the class of steroids that are the most potent of all medicines in functioning to relieve pain by reducing irritation and/or inflammation in muscles and joints.

In prescribing steroids, I use the same dose regimen employed to treat the common skin reaction to touching poison ivy leaves. If the oils from this plant have contacted much of the body, the widespread skin reaction with its accompanying severe itching can produce severe discomfort to the patient. When that is the case, use of steroids for about one week will bring the poison ivy reaction to a full stop. The problem with the steroids, in contrast to the nonsteroidal anti-inflammatories, is that they can be extremely dangerous when used for long periods. So I only try them for a one-week period, and when nothing else works. For short-term use, one need only worry about prior medical problems with stomach ulcer or tuberculosis. The steroids reactivate both of these conditions. If the patient has no history of either problem, the risk is slight.

You may wonder about the worth of a treatment that lasts for only a week. That is not the question I ask. The first question I ask is whether or not it might help. If I try this line of treatment and the patient tells me that it helped only a little, to me that means it is not worth much. But if I try it on a patient who tells me that much or even all her pain disappeared by the third day of treatment, that is important. Although such a response is not common in my experience, it does occur. Steroids are worth a try for the patient with moderate to severe pain when nothing else helps. When steroids are effective in CFS and FM patients with no obvious inflammatory component in their illness, their success makes me believe that the patient has an underlying rheumatological illness, such as lupus. Yet I have usually been unable to make that diagnosis definitively. So I continue to hold the CFS diagnosis and am glad I have found something that helps.

There are a few points to keep in mind if you are a patient whose doctor agrees to try steroids. First, if they work, the effect will probably last a lot longer than one week. Second, you may be very disappointed if your pain returns. But the very fact that the pain can be treated is therapy in itself. You, the patient, *can* feel better. Feeling better for one week is a lot better than never feeling better, and it means that you can feel better again. When steroids work, I am willing to repeat the trial after a few months have passed. If the drugs continue to be helpful, I see no problem in using them several times a year. The effect of being well is a powerful tool in convincing someone with chronic disease that good health is a possibility. Unfortunately, this outcome is rare except for the patient with the suggestion of an inflammatory component to the illness.

Other Tactics

Some patients have pain that lasts despite all these treatments. What can be done for them? The question of how to deal with chronic treatment-resistant pain is difficult. My rule is to resist using narcotics, because they often turn out to be more trouble than they are worth. Side effects of nausea, bowel disturbance, and loss of effectiveness with increased pain when they are stopped make their use questionable. When no other option remains, I will turn to them, in association with experts in pain management. When severe pain continues in the face of the treatments I have described, I often ask the patient to visit the pain clinic in our medical school for a second opinion. The pervasiveness of chronic pain is responsible for the existence of such clinics. If you live anywhere near a city, you will find one available to you. Treatments such as acupuncture and biofeedback, which are often available in pain centers, have been shown to be effective in relieving fibromyalgia pain.[20] And experts in pain management know which opiates to turn to and how to use them when needed for the CFS or FM patient whom nothing else helps.

A Role for Stimulants

The last group of medicines I try are low-dose brain stimulants, most often Ritalin or Cylert. Doctors routinely use these drugs in attention deficit disorder, in certain sleep disorders, and in depression when other medicines simply do not work. Most stimulants are in the restricted class of drugs. They have the potential for real abuse because people sometimes seek them out in order to get a chemical high. This problem, plus doctors' lack of experience in using them, are the reasons some family doctors are loath to prescribe them for severe fatigue. Still, I believe these drugs do have a role in helping the patient find *some* time during the day when severe lethargy and/or mental confusion are not pervasive. My opinion seems to be shared by other doctors who treat chronic fatigue syndrome.

A CFS discussion group for interested physicians exists on the Net; in May 1997 one topic was utilization of these agents, and nearly every respondent endorsed their careful use. Moreover, a group from the Medical College of Ohio has used this class of drugs to treat patients with posturally related fainting. Fainting while in the erect posture is probably related to the increased fatigue and dizziness that some CFS patients report when standing. The Ohio group found that Ritalin reversed tilt-test sensitivity in six of seven patients who were resistant to the medical regimen described earlier in this chapter.[21]

When I use stimulant drugs, I usually work in association with a psychiatrist who is an expert in medicines that improve mental function. These doctors are called psychopharmacologists. Their forte is drug treatment rather than psychotherapy. With the change in emphasis from psychology to biology in today's training programs in psychiatry, doctors expert in psychopharmacology are becoming easier to find. So if your doctor seems unwilling to try this class of drugs, perhaps he can work with a psychopharmacologist to determine the correct course of treatment using these agents.

Cerebral stimulants are activators and as such they have some undesirable side effects: insomnia and anxiety. To circumvent these problems, I use very low doses, most often of Ritalin or Cylert, and I give them as early in the day as is possible. Cylert is the easier for a doctor to prescribe because it is not in the restricted class of drugs.

Cylert is gentler and smoother in its action than Ritalin, but it still is the second choice. It has the potential for liver toxicity—usually only an increase in blood tests reflecting liver function. On rare occasions the drug has produced life-threatening liver disease. If you are taking this drug, your doctor must check your liver function periodically. Although it had been the perception of many doctors that Cylert was helpful in MS fatigue, a recent study[22] showed it to be no more effective than a placebo sugar pill. The only way to determine whether Cylert is really helpful in relieving the fatigue in CFS would be to do a similar double-blind study.

Ritalin is another cerebral stimulant. I believe it has a definite role in the treatment of severe fatiguing illness with mental confusion, but doctors do not like to prescribe it because it requires keeping special records and because it has a potential for abuse. Of course, I reserve this drug for patients who have had only limited benefit from my other efforts, so I prescribe it for only a relatively few of my many patients. If a patient has had a problem with substance abuse or with alcohol in the past, this drug is inappropriate.

When I do prescribe Ritalin, I first confer with my consulting psychopharmacologist and, if we agree, start with half of the normal pill size—2.5 milligrams upon awakening. If needed, I give a second 2.5 milligrams at lunch. Rarely do I need to increase dosage above a whole pill on awakening and at lunch. Since the total amount taken is small, my patients have had no abuse-type problems. About half of the patients report that it helps clear thinking and makes them feel better than they have in months. The other half report that it does not work or the side effects of nervousness or upset stomach cause them to discontinue it.

Obviously, use of either Ritalin or Cylert is not curative in any sense, but these drugs certainly give a boost to mental function and make a patient with severe and long-lasting fatigue feel better. And this kind of improvement has to be the goal of every doctor. If these medicines do not work, your doctor will have to refer you directly to the psychopharmacologist to try either stronger stimulants or combinations of medicines whose side-effect profiles are increased by their being used together. In the rare cases where our center psychopharmacologist has had to employ these methods, the few patients who have required this approach have been helped, and we have had no problem with abuse. It is self-evident that drugs in this class would never be indicated for patients who have had prior difficulties with alcohol or substance abuse.

Need for Further Drug Trials

These treatment options, in association with cognitive restructuring and gentle physical conditioning, represent the type of treatment that many experts in CFS and FM use to treat their patients. Every physician develops his or her own treatment strategy and pharmacopeia to treat illnesses such as CFS, so you can expect that your own doctor may have still other approaches. All treatments are limited by two facts: the cause(s) of CFS are not known, and a specific treatment for the illness does not exist. That is why trying drugs with different mechanisms of action is such an important research tactic.

Let me give you an example. In the late 1980s CFS was thought to be chronic Epstein-Barr disease, as I have detailed in Chapter 4. To test this idea, Steven Straus (the researcher in infectious diseases at the NIH) did a placebo-controlled treatment trial with intravenous acyclovir, an antiviral drug. The drug did not relieve the CFS symptoms. Although some infectious disease specialists still argue that acylovir is not the right drug with which to treat EBV, the negative results helped convince the scientific community that CFS was not synonymous with chronic EBV infection.

What this means is that a therapeutic trial can provide support for ideas about what causes CFS. Had the acyclovir trial been successful, it would have supported the idea that CFS was caused by a virus. That line of thinking makes the entire CFS community—patients as well as physicians—interested in Ampligen, a drug with both antiviral activity and the ability to reduce the body's immunological response to foreign substances. Ampligen was tried in a placebo-controlled study in CFS, and a small but definite improvement was seen in the functional status of the patients receiving the active drug.[23] The drug has to be given intravenously, can produce CFS-like symptoms because it itself resembles a cytokine, and is very costly. Factoring everything together, the FDA was not sufficiently impressed by the study to approve Ampligen for use in this country. The drug is available in Canada and for limited numbers of patients at several designated treatment sites in the United States, but patients in both countries have to pay many thousands of dollars for a year's supply. The company making Ampligen is currently negotiating with the FDA to start another trial in the hope of showing enough clinical improvement that the FDA will accept the drug for use in the United States. If this proposed trial upholds the value of Ampligen, it will mean that CFS— at least for some patients—has a viral or immunological cause.

Because of the large population of patients with CFS, other drug companies have medicines in the pipeline that they believe will help the CFS sufferer. In the next few years, we should be reading about these therapeutic trials. Some of them, let us hope, will reduce symptoms. This will be an obvious boon to everyone interested in severe fatiguing illness because it will give us another track to follow in understanding the cause of this debilitating illness.

13 ⟨ Summing Up

Some ends need to be tied here at the end of this book. In Chapter 5 I explained why those of you with severe fatigue may run into problems finding a physician who will listen to you and develop a rational plan for helping you. But understanding why it is hard to find a doctor does not solve the problem of actually finding one. How do you locate the right doctor for you?

Searching for the Appropriate Physician

One option is to turn to an academic center. Academic centers are usually in medical universities and staffed by exceptionally well trained physicians and ancillary medical personnel, including physical therapists and counselors of many different backgrounds. In the United States, academic physicians associated with medical centers and with expertise in fatiguing illness can be found in Newark (New Jersey Medical School), Baltimore (Johns Hopkins University), Bethesda (National Institute of Allergy and Infectious Diseases), Boston (Harvard University), Chicago (University of Illinois), Denver (University of Colorado), Harrisburg (Pennsylvania State University), Louisville (University of Louisville), Miami (University of Miami),

Portland (University of Oregon), San Francisco (University of California), Seattle (University of Washington), Stony Brook (State University of New York), and Temple (Texas A&M University). Outside the United States, academics interested in fatiguing illness may be found in Auckland, Aviano, Brussels, Dalhousie, Glasgow, Leeds, Liège, London, Moscow, Niigata, Nijmegen, Stockholm, Sydney, Tel Aviv, and Toronto.

If you do not live near one of these cities but are close to another large city, you may have to be a bit of a detective to find appropriate medical help. Large cities in every state do have academic centers, but they may not have a lot of expertise in dealing with severe fatigue. But because of the depth of medical expertise in any academic center, probably at least one physician has had a great deal of experience in caring for people with difficult medical problems. She or he could be a rheumatologist and know a lot about fibromyalgic pain, a cardiologist who cares for patients with mitral valve prolapse, a gastroenterologist with expertise in irritable bowel syndrome, an infectious disease specialist who evaluates people with repeated infections or persistent low-grade fevers, a urologist who follows many patients with interstitial cystitis, or a neurologist with a large practice devoted to headache. One of these physicians might well be able to help you—especially if they are willing to think and read about your problem.

Suppose no academic center is near you. Then you need to seek a similar large grouping of physicians where choices might be available to you. Medical economics and a work week that is too long are forcing physicians out of single-doctor practices into large physician groups. Organized medical practices consisting of several hundred doctors are common. In general, these doctors work together at the same site. But HMOs form groups of doctors often located in different sites. Again you will have to be a detective: call the administrative office of the HMO or the large physician practice to inquire about who might be the right doctor for you.

What if you do not live near such a large group of doctors or are unsuccessful as a detective? If your fatigue is very severe, you need to determine if a CFS support group exists in your area. Whether or not you want to participate in the activities of such a group is a personal decision, but they often do provide a list of physicians who are comfortable dealing with patients with fatiguing illness. If you do not live near a support group or have not found a suitable doctor, then you need to ask your personal physician for some guidance. If your problem is a persistent flu-like illness, you probably will find your way to an infectious disease specialist. If your problem is with concentration or attention, you may end up in a neurologist's office. If your problem is predominantly pain, you may see a rheumatologist.

Some of these physicians will be comfortable dealing with you, while others will not. The most common problems are that the doctor does not know much about CFS or tells you that the problem is all in your head. If the latter occurs, you need to keep looking. Such individuals are convinced that they "understand" CFS; unfortunately, such understanding does not help you. It is stigmatizing and actually could make you feel worse. If the physician either has knowledge about CFS or does not know much about it but is willing to learn about the illness, you probably have found your doctor.

Becoming Empowered

With the explosion of medical knowledge, it is impossible for any physician to keep current. When a problem arises, some doctors go to the library. Many of today's patients are better educated than those of former decades; many of you garner medical information through computer networks. Anyone can find such data on the Net, as the National Library of Medicine now provides free access to its data base of medical publications. For free MEDLINE access, type in on your Web browser:

http://www.nim.nih.gov

Many doctors tell me that their interaction with knowledgeable patients is one thing that makes the practice of medicine appealing. So bring the results of your Net search to your doctor. A doctor who welcomes your input is empowering.

Going to see a doctor with a complaint of illness that has no definite cause carries with it potential traps. Most academic physicians have my bias: they do not use unproven treatments, especially if they are at all dangerous. While most doctors would be loath to use unproven treatments that are definitely dangerous, quite a few are willing to try unproven treatments if the risk is relatively small or nonexistent. That brings you into the realm of alternative medicine. The trap there is that its practitioners also believe they understand your illness and will tell you that they can either greatly improve you or actually cure you. How do you decide whether to choose this option, and if you do, whom do you choose?

Alternative Medicine

Alternative medicine stays "alternative" to regular medicine because these therapies are not backed up by proof that they work. Until the hard research is done to prove such treatments efficacious, your decision to turn in that direction is based on your belief that they will help—not on the fact that they do work. Of course if one such treatment does not work, the next one might. That is the catch to the sufferer: you can go from one promise to the next.

You may ask about my beliefs in this matter. From my comments in Chapter 7, you can see that I keep an open mind about Asian healing practices. These have been in existence for many hundreds, even thousands, of years and I reason that time would have shown them to be valueless if indeed they were. Acupuncture is an example of an Asian medical therapy that we know is effective, at least for relieving pain. Yoga, acupuncture, and Chinese herbal medicine seem reasonable avenues to try—if my structured approach of drug therapy, gentle physical conditioning, and cognitive behavioral therapy do not sufficiently reduce your symptoms.

Beyond listing these choices, I am afraid I cannot be helpful. I know this is an important issue for many of you, but there simply is no formula for deciding which treatment to try and at what dose. Since no wave of cures has followed any of these treatments, my guess is that the majority will not make you better—at least not more than briefly. Your decision to utilize these alternative treatments depends strongly on your comfort level in trying the unknown.

One piece of advice is to question your doctor carefully about the risks of these alternative therapies. Sufficiently high doses of any drug can cause side effects, and vitamins and minerals must be viewed as drugs when they are given at high doses. So even taking vitamins has a potential risk—especially when large amounts are ingested. Any intravenous preparation carries a special risk because the drug is going directly into your bloodstream, and special diets can alter your nutritional balance. Moving away from a well-balanced "heart-healthy" diet to some alternative nutritional plan can be viewed as a stress to the body. Indeed, I worry that with underlying illness your ability to tolerate any stress—even a dietary one—could be reduced, with potentially risky side effects as the consequence of this choice.

My other advice about alternative treatments is to go out on the Internet to seek input from others who have tried such treatments. You may not be surprised at how many patients report no results from such treatment, but you may be very surprised at the host of side effects reported. If you want input on any alternative treatment, Dr. Renner's hot line is a reasonable place to turn (see Tip 2 in Chapter 10). Finally, remember my six-week rule. If you are not sure you are definitely better after six weeks of a treatment, stop and see how you feel when no longer taking it. And of course stop if you notice new symptoms developing; they could be a result of the treatment and not of your illness. The final variable to consider is cost. Despite being "natural," or "food supplements," or vitamins, alternative treatments often are costly and rarely are covered by any health insurance plan. If your disposable income is modest, I would shun this avenue.

The Quest for Feeling Better

The person suffering with severe fatigue knows only too well that there is no easy solution for the problem. Dealing with it requires hard work for you, your physician, and your coach. Even if you succeed in finding a physician and a coach who will listen to your thoughts and concerns, you will be frustrated because the "answer" just is not there. Another source of frustration is that it takes energy to cope with fatigue, and by definition energy levels are low. Sometimes the coping process may seem too much for you. Perhaps your coach and/or physician can offer you new coping strategies to reduce your frustration. Being in a true dialogue with such individuals is in itself empowering and therapeutic. Working together, the three of you will be better able to arrive at a successful formula for dealing with the frustration of unexplained illness than you could alone. Helping individuals handle this frustration is one of my prime goals in treating patients who suffer from severe and chronic fatigue.

Frustration brings demoralization along with it. So relieving frustration reduces demoralization. As demoralization lessens, strength and ability to cope return. When pain is lessened by appropriate treatment, you will again be able to take a giant step forward. Feeling better a little means that you can feel better a lot; it is only a matter of time. The wonderful clearheaded feeling that follows a bout of aerobic exercise magnifies wellness. If symptoms remain, the collaboration between you and your physician to treat each additional symptom lets you move one step at a time toward health.

Feeling better in itself is a giant step ahead. It allows you to see yourself as recovering rather than as always sick. The sense that recovery is possible allows you to begin the process of mental recovery also.

Denial and dependence lessen. It becomes easy to believe your daily mantra that you are getting better and better. The possibility of part-time work becomes real. Moving from sickness into the workplace is in itself part of the treatment. This sort of activity, even if limited, helps the chronically ill but recovering patient feel better about herself. Anything that moves the process from sickness to health is part of the treatment.

The process is very slow and for some patients virtually impossible to notice. But every patient with every illness can feel better. Becoming empowered to move in this direction has to be the goal of every sick person. Your doctor and coach can help, and the three of you together will set out the plan. The move to wellness is real. It takes effort. You can achieve it.

⟨ Resources

ℂ Notes

1. Definitions and Prevalence

1. T. L. Stedman, *Stedman's Medical Dictionary, Illustrated,* Baltimore: Williams and Wilkins, 1973.
2. G. K. Montgomery, "Uncommon Tiredness among College Undergraduates," *Journal of Consulting and Clinical Psychology* 51 (1983): 517–525.
3. National Center for Health Statistics, C. Nelson, and T. McLemore, *National Ambulatory Medical Care Survey, US: 1975–1981 and 1985 Trends,* Washington, D.C.: Government Printing Office, 1988.
4. See note 2.
5. R. Fuhrer and S. Wessely, "The Epidemiology of Fatigue and Depression: A French Primary-Care Study," *Psychological Medicine* 25 (1995): 895–905. Also G. Lewis and S. Wessely, "The Epidemiology of Fatigue: More Questions than Answers," *Journal of Epidemiology and Community Health* 46 (1992): 92–97.
6. J. R. Hughes, R. S. Crow, D. R. Jacobs, Jr., et al., "Physical Activity, Smoking, and Exercise-Induced Fatigue," *Journal of Behavioral Medicine* 7 (1984): 217–230.
7. S. Wessely, J. Nickson, and B. Cox, "Symptoms of Low Blood Pressure: A Population Study," *British Medical Journal* 301 (1990): 362–365.
8. T. Pawlikowska, T. Chalder, S. R. Hirsch, et al., "Population Based Study of Fatigue and Psychological Distress," *British Medical Journal* 304 (1994): 763–766.
9. K. Kroenke and A. D. Mangelsdorff, "Common Symptoms in Ambulatory Care: Incidence, Evaluation, Therapy, and Outcome," *American Journal of Medicine* 86 (1989): 262–266.

10. A. David, A. Pelosi, E. McDonald, et al., "Tired, Weak, or in Need of Rest: Fatigue among General Practice Attenders," *British Medical Journal* 301 (1991): 1199–1202.

11. See note 9; also P. J. Cathébras, J. M. Robbins, L. J. Kirmayer, and B. C. Hayton, "Fatigue in Primary Care: Prevalence, Psychiatric Comorbidity, Illness Behavior, and Outcome," *Journal of General Internal Medicine* 7 (1992): 276–286.

12. D. W. Bates, W. Schmitt, D. Buchwald, et al., "Prevalence of Fatigue and Chronic Fatigue Syndrome in a Primary Care Practice," *Archives of Internal Medicine* 153 (1993): 2759–65.

13. G. P. Holmes, J. E. Kaplan, N. M. Gantz, et al., "Chronic Fatigue Syndrome: A Working Case Definition," *Annals of Internal Medicine* 108 (1988): 387–389; A. Schluederberg, S. E. Straus, P. Peterson, et al., "Chronic Fatigue Syndrome Research: Definition and Medical Outcome Assessment," *Annals of Internal Medicine* 117 (1992): 325–331.

14. D. Buchwald, P. Umali, J. Umali, et al., "Chronic Fatigue and the Chronic Fatigue Syndrome: Prevalence in a Pacific Northwest Health Care System," *Annals of Internal Medicine* 123 (1995): 81–88.

15. K. Fukuda, S. E. Straus, I. Hickie, et al., "The Chronic Fatigue Syndrome: A Comprehensive Approach to Its Definition and Study," *Annals of Internal Medicine* 121 (1994): 953–959.

16. S. Wessely, T. Chalder, S. Hirsch, et al., "The Prevalence and Morbidity of Chronic Fatigue and Chronic Fatigue Syndrome: A Prospective Primary Care Study," *American Journal of Public Health* (in press).

17. P. D. White, S. A. Grover, H. O. Kangro, et al., "The Validity and Reliability of the Fatigue Syndrome That Follows Glandular Fever," *Psychological Medicine* 25 (1995): 917–924.

2. Causes of Fatigue

1. C. Wood and M. E. Magnello, "Diurnal Changes in Perceptions of Energy and Mood," *Journal of the Royal Society of Medicine* 85 (1992): 191–194.

2. J. Angst, "Epidemiology of Depression," *Psychopharmacology (Berlin)* 106 Suppl. (1992): S71–S74.

3. L. S. Radoff, "The CES-D Scale: A Self-Report Depression Scale for Research in the General Population." *Applied Psychological Measurement* 1 (1977): 385–401.

4. H. Schulberg, M. Saul, M. McClelland, et al., "Assessment of Depression in Primary Medical and Psychiatric Practices," *Archives of General Psychiatry* 42 (1985): 1164–70.

5. P. B. Beeson, "Age and Sex Associations of 40 Autoimmune Diseases," *American Journal of Medicine* 96 (1994): 457–462.

6. See note 5.

7. R. J. Dattwyler, D. J. Volkman, B. J. Luft, et al., "Seronegative Lyme Disease: Dissociation of Specific T- and B-lymphocyte Responses to *Borrelia burgdorferi*," *New England Journal of Medicine* 319 (1988): 1441–46.

8. V. Preac-Mursic, K. Weber, H. W. Pfister, et al., "Survival of Borrelia burgdorferi in Antibiotically Treated Patients with Lyme borreliosis," *Infection* 17 (1989): 355–359.

9. L. F. F. Kox, S. Kuijper, and A. H. J. Kolk, "Early Diagnosis of Tuberculous Meningitis by Polymerase Chain Reaction," *Neurology* 45 (1995): 2228–32.

10. C. Guilleminault and S. Mondini, "Mononucleosis and Chronic Daytime Sleepiness," *Archives of Internal Medicine* 146 (1986): 1333–35.

11. T. Young, M. Palta, J. Dempsey, et al., "The Occurrence of Sleep-Disordered Breathing among Middle-Aged Adults," *New England Journal of Medicine* 328 (1993): 1230–35.

12. See note 11.

13. J. E. Freal, G. H. Kraft, and J. K. Coryell, "Symptomatic Fatigue in Multiple Sclerosis," *Archives of Physical Medicine and Rehabilitation* 65 (1984): 135–138.

14. J. H. M. M. Vercoulen, O. R. Hommes, C. M. A. Swanink, et al., "The Measurement of Fatigue in Patients with Multiple Sclerosis," *Archives of Neurology* 53 (1996): 642–649.

15. R. Djaldetti, I. Ziv, A. Achiron, and E. Melamed, "Fatigue in Multiple Sclerosis Compared with Chronic Fatigue Syndrome: A Quantitative Assessment," *Neurology* 46 (1996): 632–635.

16. B. H. Natelson, J. M. Cohen, I. Brassloff, and H.-J. Lee, "A Controlled Study of Brain Magnetic Resonance Imaging in Patients with the Chronic Fatigue Syndrome," *Journal of the Neurological Sciences* 120 (1993): 213–217.

3. "Functional" Illnesses and Functional Causes of Fatigue

1. W. Calvert, D. W. Notermans, K. Staskus, et al., "Kinetics of Response in Lymphoid Tissues to Antiretroviral Therapy of HIV-1 Infection," *Science* 276 (1997): 960–964.

2. P. D. Williamson, D. D. Spencer, S. S. Spencer, et al., "Complex Partial Seizures of Frontal Lobe Origin," *Annals of Neurology* 18 (1985): 497–504.

3. S. Wessely, "Old Wine in New Bottles: Neurasthenia and 'ME'," *Psychological Medicine* 20 (1990): 35–53.

4. N. C. Ware and A. Kleinman, "Culture and Somatic Experience: The Social Course of Illness in Neurasthenia and Chronic Fatigue Syndrome," *Psychosomatic Medicine* 54 (1992): 546–560.

5. O. Paul, "Da Costa's Syndrome or Neurocirculatory Asthenia," *British Heart Journal* 58 (1987): 306–315.

6. H. Boudoulas, J. C. Reynolds, E. Mazzaferri, and C. F. Wooley, "Metabolic Studies in Mitral Valve Prolapse Syndrome: A Neuroendocrine-Cardiovascular Process," *Circulation* 61 (1980): 1200–5.

7. A. Ansari, "Syndrome of Mitral Valve Prolapse: Current Perspectives," *Progress in Cardiovascular Disease* 32 (1989): 31–72.

8. R. A. Nishimura, M. D. McGoon, C. Shub Miller, Jr., et al., "Echocardiographically Documented Mitral-Valve Prolapse: Long-term Follow-up of 237 Patients," *New England Journal of Medicine* 313 (1985): 1305–9.

9. L. C. Lum, "The Syndrome of Habitual Chronic Hyperventilation," in Q. W. Hill, ed., *Modern Trends in Psychosomatic Medicine*, pp. 727–746, London: Butterworths, 1976.

10. G. J. Magarian, "Hyperventilation Syndromes: Infrequently Recognized Common Expressions of Anxiety and Stress," *Medicine* 61 (1982): 219–236.

11. R. Fried, *The Breath Connection*, New York: Plenum Press, 1990.

12. C. Bass and W. N. Gardner, "Respiratory and Psychiatric Abnormalities in Chronic Symptomatic Hyperventilation," *British Medical Journal* 290 (1985): 1387–90.

13. See note 12.

14. J. R. Nethercott, L. L. Davidoff, B. Curbow, and H. Abbey, "Multiple Chemical Sensitivities Syndrome: Toward a Working Case Definition," *Archives of Environmental Health* 48 (1993): 19–26.

15. D. W. Black, A. Rathe, and R. B. Goldstein, "Environmental Illness: A Controlled Study of 26 Subjects with '20th Century Disease,'" *Journal of the American Medical Association* 264 (1990): 3166–70.

16. D. W. Bates, W. Schmitt, D. Buchwald, et al., "Prevalence of Fatigue and Chronic Fatigue Syndrome in a Primary Care Practice," *Archives of Internal Medicine* 153 (1993): 2759–65.

17. D. Buchwald and D. Garrity, "Comparison of Patients with Chronic Fatigue Syndrome, Fibromyalgia, and Multiple Chemical Sensitivities," *Archives of Internal Medicine* 154 (1994): 2049–53.

18. C. Bass, *Somatization: Physical Symptoms and Psychological Illness*, London: Blackwell Scientific Publications, 1990.

19. J. F. Kinzl, C. Traweger, and W. Biebl, "Family Background and Sexual Abuse Associated with Somatization," *Psychotherapy and Psychosomatics* 64 (1995): 82–87; T. K. J. Craig, A. P. Boardman, K. Mills, et al., "The South London Somatisation Study. I: Longitudinal Course and the Influence of Early Life Experiences," *British Journal of Psychiatry* 163 (1993): 579–588.

20. G. R. Smith and R. A. Monson, "Patients with Multiple Unexplained Symptoms—Their Characteristics, Functional Health, and Health Care Utilization," *Archives of Internal Medicine* 146 (1986): 69–72.

21. P. R. Slavney, *Perspectives on "Hysteria,"* Baltimore: Johns Hopkins University Press, 1990.

22. E. T. O. Slater and E. Glithero, "A Follow-up of Patients Diagnosed as Suffering from 'hysteria,'" *Journal of Psychosomatic Research* 9 (1965): 9–13.

4. Chronic Fatigue Syndrome

1. F. Wolfe, H. A. Smythe, M. B. Yunus, et al., "The American College of Rheumatology 1990 Criteria for the Classification of Fibromyalgia: Report of the Multicenter Criteria Committee," *Arthritis and Rheumatism* 33 (1990): 160–172.

2. D. L. Goldenberg, R. W. Simms, A. Geiger, and A. L. Komaroff, "High Frequency of Fibromyalgia in Patients with Chronic Fatigue Seen in a Primary Care Practice," *Arthritis and Rheumatism* 33 (1990): 381–387.

3. A. M. Ramsay, *Myalgic Encephalomyelitis and Postviral Fatigue States: The Saga of Royal Free Disease*, London: Gower Medical Publishing Co., 1988.

4. D. A. Henderson and A. Shelokov, "Epidemic Neuromyasthenia—Clinical Syndrome?" *New England Journal of Medicine* 260 (1959): 757–764.

5. G. P. Holmes, J. E. Kaplan, J. A. Stewart, et al., "A Cluster of Patients with a Chronic Mononucleosis-like Syndrome," *Journal of the American Medical Association* 257 (1987): 2297–2302.

6. R. Arav-Boger and Z. Spirer, "Chronic Fatigue Syndrome: Pediatric Aspects," *Israel Journal of Medical Sciences* 31 (1995): 330–334; S. Wessely, "Le syndrome de fatigue chronique (SFC)," *L'Encephale* 20 (1994): 581–595; M. Moutschen, J. M. Triffaux, J. Demonty, et al., "Pathogenic Tracks in Fatigue Syndromes," *Acta Clinica Belgica* 49 (1994): 274–289; A. DeLacerda, "CFS," *Jornal Brasileiro de Psiquiatria* 44 (1995): 15–18; Y. Dhein, "Erschöpfungssyndrom: ausloser ist haufig ein infekt diagnostik-ätiologie-therapie," *Fortschritte der Medizin* 113 (1995): 20–22; H. Hamre, "CFS—A Review of the Literature," *Tidsskr nor Laegeforen* 115 (1995): 3042–45; T. Kitani, "CFS," *Nippon Naika Gakkai Zasshi* 82 (1993): 1571–76; F. Rizzo, "'CFS': malattie infecttiva o psicosomatica?" *Giornale di Malattie Infecttiva e Parassitarie* 46 (1994): 724–727; M. Przewlocka, "CFS," *Polski Tygodnik Lekarski* 49 (1994): 593–595; A. Rasmussen, "Kronisk traethedssyndrom—en afgraenset enhed?" *Ugeskrift For Laeger* 156 (1994): 6832–36; and I. Zavalishin, "The CFS," *Zhurnal Nevropatologii i Psikhiatrii Imeni SS Korsakova* 94 (1994): 44–46.

7. J. F. Jones, C. G. Ray, L. L. Minnich, et al., "Evidence for Active Epstein-Barr Virus Infection in Patients with Persistent, Unexplained Illnesses: Elevated Anti–Early Antigen Antibodies," *Annals of Internal Medicine* 102 (1985): 1–7; S. E. Straus, G. Tosato, G. Armstrong, et al., "Persisting Illness and Fatigue in Adults with Evidence of Epstein-Barr Virus Infection," *Annals of Internal Medicine* 102 (1985): 7–16.

8. C. A. Horwitz, W. Henle, G. Henle, et al., "Long-term Serological Follow-up of Patients for Epstein-Barr Virus after Recovery from Infectious Mononucleosis," *Journal of Infectious Diseases* 151 (1985): 1150–53; D. Gold, R. Bowden, J. Sixbey, et al., "Chronic Fatigue: A Prospective Clinical and Virologic Study," *Journal of the American Medical Association* 264 (1990): 48–53. See also note 5.

9. G. P. Holmes, J. E. Kaplan, N. M. Gantz, et al., "Chronic Fatigue Syndrome: A Working Case Definition," *Annals of Internal Medicine* 108 (1988): 387–389; A. Schluederberg, S. E. Straus, P. Peterson, et al., "Chronic Fatigue Syndrome Research: Definition and Medical Outcome Assessment," *Annals of Internal Medicine* 117 (1992): 325–331.

10. D. W. Bates, D. Buchwald, J. Lee, et al., "A Comparison of Case Definitions of Chronic Fatigue Syndrome," *Clinical Infectious Diseases* 18 Suppl. 1 (1994): S11-S15.

11. W. Katon and J. Russo, "Chronic Fatigue Syndrome Criteria: A Critique of the Requirement for Multiple Physical Complaints," *Archives of Internal Medicine* 152 (1992): 1604–9; I. Hickie, A. Lloyd, D. Hadzi-Pavlovic, et al., "Can Chronic Fatigue Syndrome Be Defined by Distinct Clinical Features?" *Psychological Medicine* 25 (1995): 925–935.

12. K. Fukuda, S. E. Straus, I. Hickie, et al., "The Chronic Fatigue Syndrome: A Comprehensive Approach to Its Definition and Study," *Annals of Internal Medicine* 121 (1994): 953–959.

13. D. Buchwald, "Fibromyalgia and Chronic Fatigue Syndrome: Similarities and Differences," *Rheumatic Disease Clinics of North America* 22 (1996): 219–243.

14. B. H. Natelson, S. K. Johnson, J. DeLuca, et al., "Reducing Heterogeneity in Chronic Fatigue Syndrome: A Comparison with Depression and Multiple Sclerosis," *Clinical Infectious Diseases* 21 (1995): 1204–10.

15. R. Schweitzer, B. Kelly, A. Foran, et al., "Quality of Life in Chronic Fatigue Syndrome," *Social Science and Medicine* 41 (1995): 1367–72.

16. A. Wilson, I. Hickie, A. Lloyd, et al., "Longitudinal Study of Outcome of Chronic Fatigue Syndrome," *British Medical Journal* 308 (1994): 756–759.

17. C. Ray, S. Jeffries, and W. R. C. Weir, "Coping with Chronic Fatigue Syndrome: Illness Responses and Their Relationship with Fatigue, Functional Impairment and Emotional Status," *Psychological Medicine* 25 (1995): 937–945.

18. D. Bonner, M. Ron, T. Chalder et al., "Chronic Fatigue Syndrome: A Follow-up Study," *Journal of Neurology, Neurosurgery and Psychiatry* 57 (1994): 617–621; J. H. M. M. Vercoulen, C. M. A. Swanink, J. F. M. Fennis, et al., "Prognosis in Chronic Fatigue Syndrome: A Prospective Study on the Natural Course," *Journal of Neurology, Neurosurgery and Psychiatry* 60 (1996): 489–494; M. R. Clark, W. Katon, J. Russo, et al., "Chronic Fatigue: Risk Factors for

Symptom Persistence in a 2½ Year Follow-up Study," *American Journal of Medicine* 98 (1995): 187–195; D. H. Bombardier and D. Buchwald, "Outcome and Prognosis of Patients with Chronic Fatigue vs. Chronic Fatigue Syndrome," *Archives of Internal Medicine* 155 (1995): 2105–10.

19. R. Euba, T. Chalder, A. Deale, and S. Wessely, "A Comparison of the Characteristics of Chronic Fatigue Syndrome in Primary and Tertiary Care," *British Journal of Psychiatry* 168 (1996): 121–126.

20. B. D. Carter, J. F. Edwards, W. G. Kroenenberger, et al., "Case Control Study of Chronic Fatigue in Pediatric Patients," *Pediatrics* 95 (1995): 179–186; M. S. Smith, J. Mitchell, L. Corey, et al., "Chronic Fatigue in Adolescents," *Pediatrics* 88 (1991): 195–202. See also note 6.

21. C. M. A. Swanink, J. H. M. M. Vercoulen, G. Bleijenberg, et al., "Chronic Fatigue Syndrome: A Clinical and Laboratory Study with a Well Matched Control Group," *Journal of Internal Medicine* 237 (1995): 499–506; U. Tirelli, A. Pinto, G. Marotta, et al., "Clinical and Immunologic Study of 205 Patients with Chronic Fatigue Syndrome: A Case Series from Italy," *Archives of Internal Medicine* 153 (1993): 116–117; A. Hilgers, G. R. F. Krueger, U. Lembke, and A. Ramon, "Postinfectious Chronic Fatigue Syndrome: Case History of Thirty-five Patients in Germany," *In Vivo* 5 (1991): 201–206.

22. H. Kuratsune, K. Yamaguti, M. Takahashi, et al., "Acylcarnitine Deficiency in Chronic Fatigue Syndrome," *Clinical Infectious Diseases* 18 Suppl. 1 (1994): S62–S67.

23. J. G. Dobbins, B. H. Natelson, I. Brassloff, et al., "Physical, Behavioral, and Psychological Risk Factors for Chronic Fatigue Syndrome: A Central Role for Stress?" *Journal of the Chronic Fatigue Syndrome* 1 (1995): 43–58.

24. K. M. Bell, D. Cookfair, D. S. Bell, et al., "Risk Factors Associated with Chronic Fatigue Syndrome in a Cluster of Pediatric Cases," *Reviews of Infectious Diseases* 13 Suppl. 1 (1991): S32–S38.

25. A. S. Khan, W. M. Heneine, L. E. Chapman, et al., "Assessment of a Retrovirus Sequence and Other Possible Risk Factors for the Chronic Fatigue Syndrome in Adults," *Annals of Internal Medicine* 118 (1993): 241–245.

26. K. L. MacDonald, M. T. Osterholm, K. H. LeDell, et al., "A Case-control Study to Assess Possible Triggers and Cofactors in Chronic Fatigue Syndrome," *American Journal of Medicine* 100 (1996): 548–554.

27. E. Shorter, *From Paralysis to Fatigue—A History of Psychosomatic Illness in the Modern Era,* New York: Free Press, 1992; P. Manu, D. A. Matthews, and T. J. Lane, "The Mental Health of Patients with a Chief Complaint of Chronic Fatigue," *Archives of Internal Medicine* 148 (1988): 2213–17.

28. P. J. Cathébras, J. M. Robbins, L. J. Kirmayer, and B. C. Hayton, "Fatigue in Primary Care: Prevalence, Psychiatric Comorbidity, Illness Behavior, and

Outcome," *Journal of General Internal Medicine* 7 (1992): 276–286; L. Ridsdale, A. Evans, W. Jerrett, et al., "Patients with Fatigue in General Practice: A Prospective Study," *British Medical Journal* 307 (1993): 103–106; A. David, A. Pelosi, E. McDonald, et al., "Tired, Weak, or in Need of Rest: Fatigue among General Practice Attenders," *British Medical Journal* 301 (1991): 1199–1202.

29. P. Manu, T. J. Lane, and D. A. Matthews, "The Frequency of the Chronic Fatigue Syndrome in Patients with Symptoms of Persistent Fatigue," *Annals of Internal Medicine* 109 (1988): 554–556.

30. B. H. Natelson, S. P. Ellis, P. J. ÓBraonáin, et al. "Frequency of Deviant Immune Test Values in Chronic Fatigue Syndrome," *Clinical & Diagnostic Laboratory Immunology* 2 (1995): 238–240.

31. See note 14.

32. C. M. Pepper, L. B. Krupp, F. Friedberg, et al., "A Comparison of Neuropsychiatric Characteristics in Chronic Fatigue Syndrome, Multiple Sclerosis, and Major Depression," *Journal of Neuropsychiatry and Clinical Neurosciences* 5 (1993): 200–205; R. Powell, R. Dolan, and S. Wessely, "Attributions and Self-Esteem in Depression and Chronic Fatigue Syndromes," *Journal of Psychosomatic Research* 24 (1990): 665–673.

33. S. K. Johnson, J. DeLuca, and B. H. Natelson, "Depression in Fatiguing Illness: Comparing Patients with Chronic Fatigue Syndrome, Multiple Sclerosis and Depression," *Journal of Affective Disorders* 39 (1996): 21–30.

34. J. H. M. M. Vercoulen, C. M. A. Swanink, F. G. Zitman, et al., "Randomised, Double-Blind, Placebo-Controlled Study of Fluoxetine in Chronic Fatigue Syndrome," *Lancet* 347 (1996): 858–861.

35. T. J. Lane, P. Manu, and D. A. Matthews, "Depression and Somatization in the Chronic Fatigue Syndrome," *American Journal of Medicine* 91 (1991): 335–344.

36. S. K. Johnson, J. DeLuca, and B. H. Natelson, "Assessing Somatization Disorder in Chronic Fatigue Syndrome," *Psychosomatic Medicine* 58 (1996): 50–57.

37. P. Trigwell, S. Hatcher, M. Johnson, et al., " 'Abnormal' Illness Behaviour in Chronic Fatigue Syndrome and Multiple Sclerosis," *British Medical Journal* 311 (1995): 15–18.

38. P. Manu, G. Affleck, H. Tennen, et al., "Hypochondriasis Influences Quality-of-Life Outcomes in Patients with Chronic Fatigue," *Psychotherapy and Psychosomatics* 65 (1996): 76–81.

39. See note 34.

40. S. Wessely, "Old Wine in New Bottles: Neurasthenia and 'ME,' " *Psychological Medicine* 20 (1990): 35–53.

41. M. H. Lavietes, B. H. Natelson, D. L. Cordero, et al., "Does the Stressed Chronic Fatigue Syndrome Patient Hyperventilate?" *International Journal of Behavioral Medicine* 3 (1996): 70–83.

42. C. M. A. Swanink, J. W. M. Van der Meer, J. H. M. M. Vercoulen, et al., "Epstein-Barr Virus (EBV) and the Chronic Fatigue Syndrome: Normal Virus Load in Blood and Normal Immunologic Reactivity in the EBV Regression Assay," *Clinical Infectious Diseases* 20 (1995): 1390–92.
43. P. D. White, S. A. Grover, H. O. Kangro, et al., "The Validity and Reliability of the Fatigue Syndrome That Follows Glandular Fever," *Psychological Medicine* 25 (1995): 917–924.
44. D. Buchwald, P. R. Cheney, D. L. Peterson, et al., "A Chronic Illness Character-ized by Fatigue, Neurologic and Immunologic Disorders, and Active Human Herpesvirus Type 6 Infection," *Annals of Internal Medicine* 116 (1992): 103–113; M. Patnaik, A. L. Komaroff, E. Conley, et al., "Prevalence of IgM Antibodies to Human Herpesvirus 6 Early Antigen (p41/38) in Patients with Chronic Fatigue Syndrome," *Journal of Infectious Diseases* 172 (1995): 1364–67.
45. D. Di Luca, M. Zorzenon, P. Mirandola, et al., "Human Herpesvirus 6 and Human Herpesvirus 7 in Chronic Fatigue Syndrome," *Journal of Clinical Microbiology* 33 (1995): 1660–61.
46. W. J. Martin, L. C. Zeng, K. Ahmed, and M. Roy, "Cytomegalovirus-Related Sequence in an Atypical Cytopathic Virus Repeatedly Isolated from a Patient with Chronic Fatigue Syndrome," *American Journal of Pathology* 145 (1994): 440–451.
47. A. C. Mawle, M. Reyes, and D. S. Schmid, "Is Chronic Fatigue Syndrome an Infectious Disease?" *Infectious Agents and Disease* 2 (1994): 333–341.
48. G. E. Yousef, G. F. Mann, D. G. Smith, et al., "Chronic Enterovirus Infection in Patients with Postviral Fatigue Syndrome," *Lancet* 1 (1988): 146–150; N. A. Miller, H. A. Carmichael, B. D. Calder, et al., "Antibody to Coxsackie B Virus in Diagnosing Postviral Fatigue Syndrome," *British Medical Journal* 302 (1991): 140–143; C. M. A. Swanink, W. J. G. Melchers, J. W. M. Van der Meer, et al., "Enteroviruses and the Chronic Fatigue Syndrome," *Clinical Infectious Diseases* 19 (1994): 860–864.
49. J. W. Gow, W. M. H. Behan, G. B. Clements, et al., "Enteroviral RNA Se-quences Detected by Polymerase Chain Reaction in Muscle of Patients with Postviral Fatigue Syndrome," *British Medical Journal* 302 (1991): 692–696; J. W. Gow, W. M. H. Behan, K. Simpson, et al., "Studies on Enterovirus in Patients with Chronic Fatigue Syndrome," *Clinical Infectious Diseases* 18 Suppl. 1 (1994): S126–S129; A. McArdle, F. McArdle, M. J. Jackson, et al., "Investigation by Polymerase Chain Reaction of Enteroviral Infection in Pa-tients with Chronic Fatigue Syndrome," *Clinical Science* 90 (1996): 295–300.
50. T. Nakaya, H. Takahashi, Y. Nakamura, et al., "Demonstration of Borna Disease Virus RNA in Peripheral Blood Mononuclear Cells Derived from

Japanese Patients with Chronic Fatigue Syndrome," *FEBS Letters* 378 (1996): 145–149.

51. R. J. Suhadolnik, N. L. Reichenbach, P. Hitzges, et al., "Upregulation of the 2-5A Synthetase/RNase L Antiviral Pathway Associated with Chronic Fatigue Syndrome," *Clinical Infectious Diseases* 18 Suppl. 1 (1994): S96–S104.

52. C. Guilleminault and S. Mondini, "Mononucleosis and Chronic Daytime Sleepiness," *Archives of Internal Medicine* 146 (1986): 1333–35; P. D. White, J. Thomas, J. Amess, et al., "The Existence of a Fatigue Syndrome after Glandular Fever," *Psychological Medicine* 25 (1995): 907–924.

53. E. S. Asch, D. I. Bujak, M. Weiss, et al., "Lyme Disease: An Infectious and Postinfectious Syndrome," *Journal of Rheumatology* 21 (1994): 454–461.

54. M. Hotopf, N. Noah, and S. Wessely, "Chronic Fatigue and Minor Psychiatric Morbidity after Viral Meningitis: A Controlled Study," *Journal of Neurology, Neurosurgery and Psychiatry* 60 (1996): 504–509.

55. W. Strober, "Immunological Function in Chronic Fatigue Syndrome," in S. Straus, ed., *Chronic Fatigue Syndrome*, pp. 207–237, New York: Marcel Dekker, 1994. See also note 47.

56. J. DeLuca, S. K. Johnson, D. Beldowicz, and B. H. Natelson, "Neuropsychological Impairments in Chronic Fatigue Syndrome, Multiple Sclerosis, and Depression," *Journal of Neurology, Neurosurgery and Psychiatry* 58 (1995): 38–43.

57. J. DeLuca, S. K. Johnson, S. P. Ellis, and B. H. Natelson, "Cognitive Functioning Is Impaired in Patients with Chronic Fatigue Syndrome Devoid of Psychiatric Disease," *Journal of Neurology, Neurosurgery and Psychiatry* 62 (1997): 151–155.

58. B. H. Natelson, J. M. Cohen, I. Brassloff, and H.-J. Lee, "A Controlled Study of Brain Magnetic Resonance Imaging in Patients with the Chronic Fatigue Syndrome," *Journal of the Neurological Sciences* 120 (1993): 213–217.

59. M. A. Demitrack, J. K. Dale, S. E. Straus, et al., "Evidence for Impaired Activation of the Hypothalamic-Pituitary-Adrenal Axis in Patients with Chronic Fatigue Syndrome," *Journal of Clinical Endocrinology and Metabolism* 73 (1991): 1224–34.

60. N. R. McGregor, R. H. Dunstan, M. Zerbes, et al., "Preliminary Determination of a Molecular Basis to Chronic Fatigue Syndrome," *Biochemical and Molecular Medicine* 57 (1996): 73–80.

61. G. Leese, P. Chattington, W. Fraser, et al., "Short-Term Night-Shift Working Mimics the Pituitary-Adrenocortical Dysfunction in Chronic Fatigue Syndrome," *Journal of Clinical Endocrinology and Metabolism* 81 (1996): 1867–70.

62. R. M. Bennett, S. R. Clark, S. M. Campbell, and C. S. Burckhardt, "Low Levels of Somatomedin C in Patients with the Fibromyalgia Syndrome: A Possible

Link between Sleep and Muscle Pain," *Arthritis and Rheumatism* 35 (1992): 1113–16.

63. J. Bearn, T. Allain, P. Coskeran, et al., "Neuroendocrine Responses to d-Fenfluramine and Insulin-Induced Hypoglycemia in Chronic Fatigue Syndrome," *Biological Psychiatry* 37 (1995): 245–252.

64. R. H. Dunstan, M. Donohoe, W. Taylor, et al., "A Preliminary Investigation of Chlorinated Hydrocarbons and Chronic Fatigue Syndrome," *Medical Journal of Australia* 163 (1995): 294–297; P. O. Behan, "Chronic Fatigue Syndrome as a Delayed Reaction to Chronic Low Dose Organophosphate Exposure," *Journal of Environmental and Nutritional Medicine* 6 (1996): 341–350.

65. R. H. T. Edwards, J. E. Clague, H. Gibson, and T. Helliwell, "Muscle Metabolism, Histopathology and Physiology in Chronic Fatigue Syndrome," in S. Straus, ed., *Chronic Fatigue Syndrome*, pp. 241–261, New York: Marcel Dekker, 1994.

66. K. K. McCully, B. H. Natelson, S. Iotti, et al., "Reduced Oxidative Muscle Metabolism in Chronic Fatigue Syndrome," *Muscle and Nerve* 19 (1996): 621–625.

67. See note 61.

68. I. Bou-Holaigah, P. C. Rowe, J. Kan, and H. Calkins, "The Relationship between Neurally Mediated Hypotension and the Chronic Fatigue Syndrome," *Journal of the American Medical Association* 274 (1995): 961–967.

69. See note 17.

70. S. Wessely and M. Sharpe, "Chronic Fatigue, Chronic Fatigue Syndrome, and Fibromyalgia," in R. Mayou, C. Bass, and M. Sharp, eds., *Treatment of Functional Somatic Symptoms*, pp. 285–312, London: Oxford University Press, 1995.

71. T. Pawlikowska, T. Chalder, S. R. Hirsch, et al., "Population Based Study of Fatigue and Psychological Distress," *British Medical Journal* 304 (1994): 763–766.

72. F. Wolfe, "The Future of Fibromyalgia: Some Critical Issues," *Journal of Musculoskeletal Pain* 3 (1995): 3–15.

5. Understanding the Doctor

1. B. H. Natelson, *Tomorrow's Doctors: The Path to Successful Practice in the 1990s*, New York: Plenum Publishing Corporation, 1990.

2. R. V. Woodward, D. H. Broom, and D. G. Legge, "Diagnosis in Chronic Illness: Disabling or Enabling—The Case of Chronic Fatigue Syndrome," *Journal of the Royal Society of Medicine* 88 (1995): 325–329.

3. S. R. Hahn, K. S. Thompson, T. A. Wills, et al., "The Difficult Doctor-Patient Relationship: Somatization, Personality and Psychopathology," *Journal of Clinical Epidemiology* 47 (1994): 647–657.

6. Problems with Sleep

1. A. B. Dollins, I. V. Zhdanova, R. J. Wurtman, et al., "Effect of Inducing Nocturnal Serum Melatonin Concentrations in Daytime on Sleep, Mood, Body Temperature, and Performance," *Proceedings of the National Academy of Sciences of the United States of America* 91 (1994): 1824–28.
2. M. Undén and B. R. Schechter, "Next Day Effects after Nighttime Treatment with Zolpidem: A Review," *European Psychiatry* 11 (suppl 1) (1996): 21s–30s.

7. The Role of Exercise in Reducing Stress

1. P. J. O'Connor, C. X. Bryant, J. P. Veltri, and S. M. Gebhardt, "State Anxiety and Ambulatory Blood Pressure following Resistance Exercise in Females," *Medicine and Science in Sports and Exercise* 25 (1993): 516–521.
2. S. Sisto, J. LaManca, D. L. Cordero, et al., "Metabolic and Cardiovascular Effects of a Progressive Exercise Test in Patients with Chronic Fatigue Syndrome," *American Journal of Medicine* 100 (1996): 634–640.
3. G. A. McCain, D. A. Bell, F. M. Mai, and P. D. Halliday, "A Controlled Study of the Effects of a Supervised Cardiovascular Fitness Training Program on the Manifestations of Primary Fibromyalgia," *Arthritis and Rheumatism* 31 (1988): 1135–41.
4. K. Y. Fulcher and P. White, "Randomised Controlled Trial of Graded Exercise in Patients with CFS," *British Medical Journal* 314 (1997): 1647–1652.
5. S. Sisto, W. N. Tapp, S. D. Drastal, et al., "Vagal Tone Is Decreased during Paced Breathing in Patients with the Chronic Fatigue Syndrome," *Clinical Autonomic Research* 5 (1995): 139–143.
6. M. Sakakibara and J. Hayano, "Effect of Slowed Respiration on Cardiac Parasympathetic Response to Threat," *Psychosomatic Medicine* 58 (1996): 32–37.
7. D. Shannahoff-Khalsa and Y. Bhajan, "The Healing Power of Sound: Techniques from Yogic Medicine," in R. Spintge and R. Droh, eds., *MusicMedicine*, pp. 179–193, St. Louis: MMB Music, 1992.

9. Help from a Coach or Consultant

1. A. Ellis and W. Dryden, "The General Theory of RET," *The Practice of Rational-Emotive Therapy (RET)*, pp. 1–27, New York: Springer Publishing Company, 1990.
2. A. T. Beck and G. Emery, *Anxiety Disorders and Phobias: A Cognitive Perspective*, New York: Basic Books, 1985; D. D. Burns, *Feeling Good: The New Mood Therapy*, New York: Signet, 1980.
3. M. Sharpe, K. Hawton, S. Simkin, et al., "Cognitive Behaviour Therapy for the Chronic Fatigue Syndrome: A Randomised Controlled Trial," *British Medical Journal* 312 (1996): 22–26; A. Deale, T. Chalder, I. Marks, and S. Wessely,

"Cognitive Behavior Therapy for Chronic Fatigue Syndrome: A Randomised Controlled Trial," *American Journal of Psychiatry* 154 (1997): 408–414.

4. J. H. M. M. Vercoulen, C. M. A. Swanink, J. F. M. Fennis, et al., "Prognosis in Chronic Fatigue Syndrome: A Prospective Study on the Natural Course," *Journal of Neurology, Neurosurgery and Psychiatry* 60 (1996): 489–494.

5. F. Friedberg and L. B. Krupp, "A Comparison of Cognitive Behavioral Treatment for Chronic Fatigue Syndrome and Primary Depression," *Clinical Infectious Diseases* 18(Suppl 1) (1994): S105–S110.

10. Tips for the Patient

1. U. Vollmer-Conna, I. Hickie, D. Hadzi-Pavlovic, et al., "Intravenous Immunoglobulin Is Ineffective in the Treatment of Patients with Chronic Fatigue Syndrome," *American Journal of Medicine* 103 (1997): 38–43.

2. G. Caplan, "Mastery of Stress: Psychosocial Aspects," *American Journal of Psychiatry* 138 (1988): 413–420.

11. The Medical Treatment of Psychological Causes of Fatigue

1. K. Rickels, R. Downing, E. Schweizer, and H. Hassman, "Antidepressants for the Treatment of Generalized Anxiety Disorder: A Placebo-Controlled Comparison of Imipramine, Trazodone, and Diazepam," *Archives of General Psychiatry* 50 (1993): 884–895.

2. J. H. M. M. Vercoulen, C. M. A. Swanink, F. G. Zitman, et al., "Randomised, Double-Blind, Placebo-Controlled Study of Fluoxetine in Chronic Fatigue Syndrome," *Lancet* 347 (1996): 858–861; F. Wolfe, M. A. Cathey, and D. J. Hawley, "A Double-Blind Placebo Controlled Trial of Fluoxetine in Fibromyalgia," *Scandinavian Journal of Rheumatology* 23 (1994): 255–259.

3. See note 2.

12. The Medical Treatment of Chronic Fatiguing Illnesses

1. K. Fukuda, S. E. Straus, I. Hickie, et al., "The Chronic Fatigue Syndrome: A Comprehensive Approach to Its Definition and Study," *Annals of Internal Medicine* 121 (1994): 953–959.

2. I. M. Cox, M. J. Campbell, and D. Dowson, "Red Blood Cell Magnesium and Chronic Fatigue Syndrome," *Lancet* 337 (1991): 757–760.

3. P. O. Behan and W. M. H. Behan, "Essential Fatty Acids in the Treatment of Postviral Fatigue Syndrome," in D. F. Horrobin, ed., *Omega 6 Essential Fatty Acids: Pathophysiology and Role in Clinical Medicine*, pp. 275–282, New York: Wiley-Liss, 1990.

4. J. Herbert, "The Age of Dehydroepiandrosterone," *Lancet* 345 (1995): 1193–94; A. J. Morales, J. J. Nolan, J. C. Nelson, and S. S. C. Yen, "Effects of Replace-

ment Dose of Dehydroepiandrosterone in Men and Women of Advancing Age," *Journal of Clinical Endocrinology and Metabolism* 78 (1994): 1360–67.

5. I. Bou-Holaigah, P. C. Rowe, J. Kan, and H. Calkins, "The Relationship between Neurally Mediated Hypotension and the Chronic Fatigue Syndrome," *Journal of the American Medical Association* 274 (1995): 961–967.

6. P. A. Low, "Update on the Evaluation, Pathogenesis and Management of Neurogenic Orthostatic Hypotension," *Neurology* 45 (Suppl. 5) (1995): S4–S32.

7. W. N. Kapoor and N. Brant, "Evaluation of Syncope by Upright Tilt Testing with Isoproterenol: A Nonspecific Test," *Annals of Internal Medicine* 116 (1992): 358–363.

8. See note 6.

9. J. H. M. M. Vercoulen, C. M. A. Swanink, F. G. Zitman, et al., "Randomised, Double-Blind, Placebo-Controlled Study of Fluoxetine in Chronic Fatigue Syndrome," *Lancet* 347 (1996): 858–861.

10. F. Wolfe, M. A. Cathey, and D. J. Hawley, "A Double-Blind Placebo Controlled Trial of Fluoxetine in Fibromyalgia," *Scandinavian Journal of Rheumatology* 23 (1994): 255–259.

11. S. Stoll, U. Hafner, O. Pohl, and W. E. Müller, "Age-Related Memory Decline and Longevity under Treatment with Selegiline," *Life Sciences* 55 (1994): 2155–63.

12. D. Goldenberg, M. Mayskiy, C. Mossey, et al., "A Randomized, Double-Blind Crossover Trial of Fluoxetine and Amitriptyline in the Treatment of Fibromyalgia," *Arthritis and Rheumatism* 39 (1996): 1852–59.

13. D. L. Goldenberg, D. T. Felson, and H. Dinerman, "A Randomized, Controlled Trial of Amitriptyline and Naproxen in the Treatment of Patients with Fibromyalgia," *Arthritis and Rheumatism* 29 (1986): 1371–77.

14. L. B. Krupp, P. K. Coyle, C. Doscher, et al., "Fatigue Therapy in Multiple Sclerosis: Results of a Double-Blind, Randomized, Parallel Trial of Amantidine, Pemoline, and Placebo," *Neurology* 45 (1995): 1956–61.

15. M. L. Cohen and J. L. Quintner, "Fibromyalgia Syndrome, A Problem of Tautology," *Lancet* 342 (1993): 906–909; G. Granges and G. Littlejohn, "Pressure Pain Threshold in Pain-Free Subjects, in Patients with Chronic Regional Pain Syndromes, and in Patients with Fibromyalgia Syndrome," *Arthritis and Rheumatism* 36 (1993): 642–646.

16. D. J. Clauw and P. Katz, "The Overlap between Fibromyalgia and Inflammatory Rheumatic Disease: When and Why Does It Occur?" *Journal of Clinical Rheumatology* 1 (1995): 335–341.

17. G. D. Middleton, J. E. McFarlin, and P. E. Lipsky, "Hydroxychloroquine and Pain Thresholds," *Arthritis and Rheumatism* 38 (1995): 445–446.

18. M. A. Demitrack, J. K. Dale, S. E. Straus, et al., "Evidence for Impaired Activation of the Hypothalamic-Pituitary-Adrenal Axis in Patients with Chronic Fatigue Syndrome," *Journal of Clinical Endocrinology and Metabolism* 73 (1991): 1224–34.

19. S. Clark, E. Tindall, and R. M. Bennett, "A Double Blind Crossover Trial of Prednisone versus Placebo in the Treatment of Fibrositis," *Journal of Rheumatology* 12 (1985): 980–983.

20. C. Deluze, L. Bosia, A. Zirbs, et al., "Electro-Acupuncture in Fibromyalgia: Results of a Controlled Trial," *British Medical Journal* 305 (1992): 1249–52; G. Ferraccioli, L. Ghirelli, F. Scita, et al., "EMG-Biofeedback Training in Fibromyalgia Syndrome," *Journal of Rheumatology* 14 (1987): 820–825.

21. B. R. Grubb, D. Kosinski, A. Mouhaffel, et al., "The Use of Methylphenidate in the Treatment of Refractory Neurocardiogenic Syncope," *Pacing and Clinical Electrophysiology* 19 (1996): 836–840.

22. See note 14.

23. D. R. Strayer, W. A. Carter, I. Brodsky, et al., "A Controlled Clinical Trial with a Specifically Configured RNA Drug, poly(I)•poly(C_{12}U), in Chronic Fatigue Syndrome," *Clinical Infectious Diseases* 18 Suppl. 1 (1994): S88–S95.

⟨ Index